AMERICAN DIABETES ASSOCIATION

GUIDE TO
RAISING
A CHILD
WITH DIABETES

SECOND EDITION

Linda M. Siminerio
RN, PhD, CDE

Jean Betschart
MN, MSN, CPNP, CDE

Director, Book Publishing, John Fedor; *Editor,* Laurie Guffey; *Production Manager,* Peggy M. Rote; *Composition,* Harlowe Typography, Inc.; *Cover Design,* Wickham & Associates, Inc.; *Printer,* Transcontinental Printing, Inc.

Printed in Canada
1 3 5 7 9 10 8 6 4 2

The suggestions and information contained in this publication are generally consistent with the *Clinical Practice Recommendations* and other policies of the American Diabetes Association, but they do not represent the policy or position of the Association or any of its boards or committees. Reasonable steps have been taken to ensure the accuracy of the information presented. However, the American Diabetes Association cannot ensure the safety or efficacy of any product or service described in this publication. Individuals are advised to consult a physician or other appropriate health care professional before undertaking any diet or exercise program or taking any medication referred to in this publication. Professionals must use and apply their own professional judgment, experience, and training and should not rely solely on the information contained in this publication before prescribing any diet, exercise, or medication. The American Diabetes Association—its officers, directors, employees, volunteers, and members—assumes no responsibility or liability for personal or other injury, loss, or damage that may result from the suggestions or information in this publication.

♾ The paper in this publication meets the requirements of the ANSI Standard Z39.48-1992 (permanence of paper).

ADA titles may be purchased for business or promotional use or for special sales. For information, please write to Lee Romano Sequeira, Special Sales & Promotions, at the address below.

American Diabetes Association
1701 North Beauregard Street
Alexandria, Virginia 22311

Library of Congress Cataloging-in-Publication Data
Siminerio, Linda M.
   American Diabetes Association guide to raising a child with diabetes / Linda Siminerio, Jean Betschart.—2nd ed.
      p. cm.
   Rev. ed. of: Raising a child with diabetes. 1995.
   Includes index.
   ISBN 1-58040-027-2 (pbk. : alk. paper)
      1. Diabetes in children—Popular works. 2. Diabetes in children—Patients—Home care.
I. Title: Guide to raising a child with diabetes. II. Betschart, Jean. III. Siminerio, Linda
M. Raising a child with diabetes. IV. Title.

RJ420.D5 S57 2000
618.92'462—dc21   00-036209

*Linda dedicates this book
to the loving memory of her father,
John A. Mulac*

*Jean dedicates this book
to the loving memory of her daughter,
Julie*

Contents

Preface

For most folks, parenthood is a challenge all by itself. Our fast-paced life today leaves little room for normal childhood issues, and when your child develops diabetes, adding the tasks of diabetes care to normal parenting responsibilities can be a huge burden of responsibility. This book is intended to help give you support and information so that you will be prepared to handle issues that come up in the daily life of your child.

Help can come from many sources: loving friends and relatives; a strong, caring medical team; and the knowledge you gather as you learn as much as you possibly can about diabetes. As your child grows and changes, the way diabetes affects her life will change as well.

The best diabetes care is flexible and dynamic. You should be able to fit your routine into the rigors of everyday life, and modify it as your child grows and develops. Food likes and dislikes come and go. Children pick up different hobbies and sports. Your approach to diabetes care will need to change based on the needs of your child, the philosophy of your health care team, and your own parenting style.

Therefore, use the guidance here in conjunction with the advice of your health care providers. There are many successful ways to treat diabetes; if you are currently doing something different from what is recommended here, it does not mean that one way is right or the other wrong. The *right* approach is the one that works best for your child and your family. And sometimes the only way of knowing which approach is best is to try several different strategies.

Two notes: we have alternated the use of he and she by chapters to avoid having to repeat the awkward "he or she" when referring to your child. Also, any mention of a brand name product does not imply endorsement of the product by the American Diabetes Association or us. We use brand names only as examples of the kinds of products available.

We are indebted to the work of Adele Faber and Elaine Mazlish and found their book, *How to Talk So Kids Will Listen & Listen So Kids Will Talk,* invaluable to us both as parents and educators.

We extend special thanks to our families for their constant support of our endeavors to promote diabetes care, to the members of the Children's Hospital of Pittsburgh Diabetes Care Team for their encouragement, and to the American Diabetes Association for their pursuit of excellence.

Linda Siminerio
Jean Betschart

Introduction

When you learn that your child has diabetes, you may feel as if your world has turned upside down. There is too much information to absorb and many questions that don't have good answers. Since insulin was first discovered around 1921, education has been a cornerstone of diabetes treatment. The more you and your child know about diabetes and how to treat it, the better equipped you will be to make decisions. This book will help you and your family learn about diabetes, and give you a framework for learning even more.

Parents commonly feel some responsibility and guilt over their child's development of diabetes. Good parenting, in most cases, means protecting your child from harm; keeping her safe. We buy special car seats, learn how to position our children in their cribs, are aware of what they put in their mouths, are careful about foods, insert protectors into electrical outlets, take them for immunizations, and watch their every move. All of these efforts are intended to control the environment and prevent anything harmful from happening to our children. So when a child develops a chronic illness which as yet has no cure, it's common to ask yourself what you could have done to prevent it.

Accept that there was *nothing* you could have done to prevent the onset of your child's diabetes. You will need to find a firm footing, dig in, and make the best of things without feeling paralyzing guilt. Even if you had known that your child was genetically at risk for diabetes, there is currently no proven way of preventing the disease from occurring. Other guilt-laden issues sometimes also arise. How do you focus on one family member when there are others who also demand your time and attention?

Your life won't ever be normal in the way it was before your child's diabetes. In time, however, you'll achieve a different kind of normality—one that includes blood test strips, emergency supplies of orange juice, syringes, and all the other paraphernalia of life with diabetes.

Diabetes can be a very unpredictable disease. You can do everything right, follow all the instructions from your doctor and dietitian, and your child's blood glucose may still not be where you want it to be. On the other hand, things may go well when you least expect them to, such as when your child is off his schedule.

Research is moving forward to find a cure, but it isn't there yet. Diabetes can't be cured—yet. But it can be controlled. New and better kinds of insulin are available. Easy-to-use glucose meters make it possible for children to check their own blood glucose levels quickly and easily. New knowledge gained from research tells us that diabetes treatment can be flexible—that rigid diets and schedules are not always necessary.

The good news is that you and your child *can* successfully adjust to life with diabetes. With knowledge, determination, and diligent medical care, your child with diabetes should be able to lead a life that is healthy, active, and happy.

What Is Diabetes?

Diabetes mellitus is not a new disorder. It was around as early as 30 A.D. Diabetes is a Greek word that means "to run through." Mellitus is a Latin word that means "honeyed." Healers coined this term to describe what they saw: people with diabetes urinated a lot and their urine was sweet.

We now know that diabetes occurs when the body cannot use and store food properly. The food we eat is made up of protein, carbohydrates, and fats. Food is broken down during digestion for the body to use for energy. Proteins are broken down into amino acids. Carbohydrates become glucose. Fats become fatty acids. These substances enter your bloodstream and travel throughout your body to feed your cells.

Glucose is the body's main energy source. But before it can be used as energy, glucose must enter the body's cells. Insulin is like a key that opens doors on the cell wall to let glucose in.

In people with diabetes, either the body does not make any or enough insulin, or it cannot use the insulin "keys" available. As a result, instead of entering the cells, glucose stays in the blood. The cells starve, and glucose levels in the blood rise. A high glucose level in the blood (also known as hyperglycemia) is a sign of diabetes.

The two most common types of diabetes are type 1 and type 2 diabetes. In type 1 diabetes, the body doesn't make enough insulin. People with this type of diabetes depend on daily injections of insulin to survive. Most children have type 1 diabetes, but adults may get it too.

Diabetes is one of the most common chronic diseases in children. Type 1 diabetes is the third most common chronic disease of childhood after asthma and mental retardation, affecting 0.5–1% of the general population during the life span. In the United States, the reported rates are between 2 and 3 children per 1,000. Every year, at least 60,000 children are diagnosed worldwide. Despite recent progress in our understanding of the genetics and immune process of the disease, diabetes continues to increase by a rate of 3–5% per year. Every year about 13,000 new cases of type 1 diabetes are diagnosed in people under 20 years of age.

In type 2 diabetes, the body makes insulin but doesn't use it properly. Although type 2 diabetes mostly affects adults, it can occur in children. Many of the signs of high blood glucose are the same in both type 1 and type 2 diabetes. People with type 2 diabetes often can manage their diabetes by watching the quantity and type of food they eat or by taking a pill, which helps them use the insulin they make more efficiently. Often, they also need to take insulin.

In the past, type 1 diabetes was called juvenile-onset and type 2 was known as maturity-onset diabetes. These names were changed because they were misleading. This book is mainly about type 1 diabetes. However, many areas of care for type 1 and type 2 diabetes are the same. A section on type 2 diabetes is included in this book (see page 96) that addresses the differences and special needs of the child with type 2 diabetes, since it is becoming more common.

THE PANCREAS

To understand type 1 diabetes you need to know about the pancreas, a large gland located behind the stomach.

The pancreas has two main jobs in the body. It makes digestive juices and chemicals called enzymes that help the body to break down food for use as fuel. The pancreas also makes hormones that help to deliver fuel to cells. One of these hormones is insulin, which helps to deliver glucose to cells.

Clusters of cells in the pancreas called the islets of Langerhans contain *beta cells*, which make insulin. Type 1 diabetes occurs when the beta cells stop making insulin. This process can be gradual or abrupt. Without insulin, the body cannot use glucose for energy. Insulin injections replace the missing insulin and allow the body to use glucose.

CAUSES OF TYPE 1 DIABETES

The reasons why the beta cells stop making insulin are not well understood. However, it is known that the destruction is due to an autoimmune process. This means that antibodies are produced, which destroy the beta cells that make insulin.

An autoimmune illness is one where the body rejects and destroys its own cells, almost like having an allergy to yourself. This process is called an *autoimmune response* and may be triggered by a virus. When the beta cells are destroyed, the pancreas can no longer make insulin and diabetes develops.

Many children who get diabetes do so shortly after having a viral illness. The peak months for the diagnosis of diabetes in children are September, January, and February, paralleling cold and flu season. The virus may have caused the autoimmune response, or the children may have been going to get diabetes anyway, and the viral illness brought it on quickly. A virus alone is almost certainly not enough to cause diabetes. Thousands of children get viral infections every year, and only a few of them get diabetes.

Scientists don't know exactly how a virus might lead to diabetes. However, they do know that some people inherit a higher risk for type 1 diabetes. People often wonder why in some families more than one person has diabetes. The reason is that in those families, family members share the genes that make them prone to diabetes.

Genes alone do not seem to cause type 1 diabetes, but they do determine your risk of getting it. It's possible that in people whose genes make them prone to diabetes, a virus or other stressor somehow flips the switch that turns on diabetes.

Some people, especially children, worry that they can "catch" diabetes from contact with someone who has it. *Diabetes is not contagious. It cannot be transmitted from one person to another.*

SIGNS AND SYMPTOMS OF DIABETES

The symptoms of diabetes are caused by blood glucose levels that are too high (*hyperglycemia*). When the body stops making insulin and high blood glucose is not treated with insulin, *ketoacidosis* may develop. Ketoacidosis is a very serious condition.

Hyperglycemia (High Blood Glucose)

Here's what happens: after food is eaten, the digestive process breaks it down into glucose. Normally, insulin helps to move glucose from the blood into the body's cells. When there is not enough insulin, glucose cannot get into the cells. The cells then begin to starve and glucose builds up in the blood. Blood glucose levels can go too high when:

▮ the body gets too little insulin, too much food, or too little exercise
▮ the body is under physical stress from a cold, sore throat, or other illness
▮ your child is feeling emotional stress

The body is always working toward a state of balance. When there is an emergency state in one system, other systems go into action to help. When the cells are starving, this is an emergency state. When your child develops diabetes, she may have some or all of the following signs and symptoms that indicate her blood glucose level is too high. Some of the following are emergency state symptoms.

■ **Frequent urination.** When your child has diabetes, high glucose in the blood filters into the urine, pulling water with it. This creates a large volume of urine and makes your child urinate a lot.

■ **Excessive thirst.** As sugar and water are pulled into the urine, dehydration begins and thirst develops. You may notice that your child becomes extremely thirsty.

■ **Weight loss.** Your child may lose weight because the body, unable to make proper use of food, tries to get nourishment by burning stored fat for energy. Weight loss also occurs due to dehydration. because the body is losing so much water in urine.

■ **Increased appetite.** This is the body's way of asking for the food it needs to gain weight and replace the calories lost in urine.

■ **Tiredness and weakness.** Your child may feel tired and weak because the body's cells are dehydrated and starving. Muscle cramping may occur. Muscles and other tissues are depleted of glucose and water.

■ **Vision problems.** Your child may complain of difficulty seeing the chalkboard or reading signs at a distance. High blood glucose can cause the lens of the eye to change shape, leading to blurred vision. This does not cause permanent eye damage. Once her blood glucose is under control, your child's vision will improve.

You will learn to recognize the signs and symptoms of hyperglycemia in your child. (For how to prevent and treat hyperglycemia, see page 84.)

Ketoacidosis and Diabetic Coma

As the signs and symptoms of high blood glucose progress and worsen, the body literally begins to starve to death. Your child can slip into a condition known as diabetic ketoacidosis or DKA. If your child did not have these signs and symptoms when she was initially diagnosed, the most likely time to see them would be during an illness, or if insulin has been omitted. Your child will appear quite ill as symptoms worsen.

Without insulin, glucose cannot enter the body's cells to provide energy. The cells are forced to burn fat to get the energy they need. When fat is burned, by-products called *ketones* build up in the blood and spill into the urine.

Small amounts of ketones are probably not harmful. However, when ketones build up they cause the blood to turn acidic, which can act like a poison. A high level of ketones in the blood and urine is called ketoacidosis. The most common causes of ketoacidosis are:

▌ undiagnosed or newly diagnosed diabetes
▌ illness
▌ too little insulin to meet the body's needs

Ketoacidosis usually does not develop without warning. The signs and symptoms of ketoacidosis are:

▌ ketones in the urine and blood
▌ dehydration (symptoms include sunken eyes; dry, cracked lips; dry mouth; and skin that remains pinched up after it is pinched)
▌ nausea and vomiting
▌ fruity-smelling breath
▌ rapid or heavy breathing
▌ abdominal pain
▌ drowsiness

If your child develops any of these symptoms, it's extremely important to contact your doctor right away. If left untreated, ketoacidosis can lead to a coma, brain swelling, and even death. However, a person can have ketoacidosis without being in a coma. With prompt treatment, children usually recover from ketoacidosis without any aftereffects at all. (For more on preventing and treating ketoacidosis, see page 86.)

Hypoglycemia (Low Blood Glucose)

Hypoglycemia is a common side effect of treatment in children with diabetes. Low blood glucose occurs when your child takes too much insulin, hasn't eaten enough food (or has eaten late), or has exercised more than usual.

When blood glucose starts to drop too low, adrenaline (a hormone that helps the body deal with emergencies) jumps into action to try to raise it. When this happens, your child may show the following signs and symptoms, which are related to this rush of adrenaline:

■ pale, clammy skin
■ sweating
■ rapid pulse
■ shakiness
■ tingling
■ hunger

Most of the time hypoglycemia is mild and can be easily treated by giving your child a sweet food. In severe hypoglycemia, the brain is deprived of glucose, causing the following symptoms:

■ headache
■ personality changes
■ irritability, crying
■ poor coordination
■ dizziness
■ confusion
■ nightmares
■ fatigue, sleepiness, unconsciousness
■ seizures

Just as you will learn to recognize the symptoms of high blood glucose in your child, you will also learn to recognize the symptoms of low blood glucose. (For how to prevent and treat hypo-glycemia, see page 80.)

KEEPING BLOOD GLUCOSE IN A TARGET RANGE

For a person without diabetes, a normal blood glucose range is between 70–120 mg/dl. Of course, it would be great if people with diabetes could always keep their blood glucose in the normal range. Although we now know that keeping blood glucose levels close to normal helps to prevent the complications of diabetes, it is very difficult to always maintain a normal level when insulin is given rather than made within one's own pancreas. If we aim at a normal blood glucose range of 70–120 mg/dl, we also run the risk of low blood glucose. Too many hypoglycemic episodes can be uncomfortable and even dangerous for children.

Therefore, it is a good idea to have a target range for your child's blood glucose level. This is the range of blood glucose levels to aim for. Decide what your child's blood glucose target should be with your child (if he's old enough) and your health care provider. You should all come to an agreement on what is reasonable and achievable to shoot for.

Just like a real target, sometimes you will hit the bull's eye and other times you will go outside of the target area. This is bound to happen. Sometimes you will know why your child's blood glucose was out of range and other times you won't. If you can't figure it out, it's okay. Sometimes blood glucose bounces and no one exactly knows why, especially in children.

Years ago, people with diabetes did not have the tools they needed to control their condition well. But now people with diabetes can do things that make diabetes easier to control, like frequently checking their blood glucose levels. Some of the new glucose meters are so easy to use that a young child can learn to do her own tests, although supervision is still essential.

In the past, people with diabetes were advised to stick to a rigid diet where all food was weighed and measured. Now, however, we know that diabetes can be successfully managed with a flexible approach to eating. There are still guidelines and structure to the meal plans, but your child can eat a variety of foods, including some with sugar. Balancing food, insulin, and exercise; testing glucose regularly; and making adjustments when necessary will help your child include special treats in her meal plan.

What's more, a meal plan that's healthy for your child with diabetes is healthy for your whole family. That means everyone can eat the same meals.

Science has created new products that make diabetes easier to manage. With artificial sweeteners, children with diabetes can enjoy sweet-tasting foods and drinks without raising blood glucose too high. New kinds of insulin have been developed that are much less likely to cause allergic reactions than those of the past and are very fast acting. Shorter, thinner needles, pen devices, and insulin pumps help make giving injections easier. It still takes energy and motivation to keep on top of diabetes management, but with education and support, you and your child will learn to live successfully with diabetes.

You and your child will most likely have good days and challenging days. Of course, you will get frustrated at times. Diabetes can be unpredictable. Sometimes things may not go well even when you do everything right. On the other hand, glucose levels may stay in range when you don't expect them to, such as on a day when your child has a party or her usual schedule is disrupted. A problem-solving approach to diabetes management is important for you and your child. If you can figure out what caused the unusual high or low, you may be able to prevent it the next time. Understanding how diabetes works in your child can help to give you the confidence you need to try to solve problems as they arise.

Caring for Your Child with Diabetes

The constant rigors of having a child with diabetes are difficult for most parents. Having diabetes can affect many aspects of your child's life and your life as a family. Most of the day-to-day care of a child with diabetes is carried out by family members and by the child when he is old enough. In many cases, the burden of care falls on one parent. It is usually best to decide as a family how to share responsibilities between family members so that no one person is overloaded. If you are a single parent, you may want to try to enlist help from friends, neighbors, other family members, churches, or intergenerational groups.

When you are deciding on a plan of care with your health care provider, it is important to take into account your child's personality, likes and dislikes, and habits. No two children with diabetes are alike or can be treated in exactly the same way. It is also important that diabetes care fits into your family's life, as well as your child's school schedule and social life, not the other way around. Although many parents at times feel enslaved to the diabetes schedule, most of the time diabetes care should fit quietly into your daily routines.

Each child with diabetes will have a treatment plan designed for him and his family's schedule. The goal of treatment is to keep your child's blood glucose levels within a target range by balancing insulin with food and exercise. A treatment plan should include:

- insulin injections
- blood glucose testing
- meal planning

Your health care professional will also be evaluating:

- treatment of high and low blood glucose levels
- your child's growth and development
- your child's success with friends, sports, school, and emotional state
- the whole family's ability to cope with life with diabetes

NEW THINKING ABOUT TREATING CHILDREN WITH DIABETES

One of the difficulties in treating diabetes in children today has been that there is little agreement about treatment and blood glucose goals in children throughout the world. It is generally agreed, however, that a child's blood glucose should be as close to normal as possible without frequent or severe hypoglycemia. How that happens in terms of treatment is widely different from one setting to another, and even one physician to another in the same setting. That can be a good thing, because diabetes care must be individualized.

Several years ago a very large, ten-year study ended that changed the direction of diabetes care. It was called the Diabetes Control and Complications Trial (DCCT). Young children did not take part in the DCCT (the participants were all between the ages of 13 and 39). Because none of the study volunteers was a child, we can't say for sure whether the study's results apply to children. However, this very important study clearly showed that keeping blood glucose levels normal or as close to normal as possible can postpone or prevent complications that are caused by diabetes.

People achieved these blood glucose levels through close supervision by a medical team, multiple daily injections or an insulin pump, careful meal planning, meticulous attention to monitoring, and frequent adjustments.

Diabetes health care providers agree that improving blood glucose control is good for everyone with diabetes, including children. Complications occur very rarely in children, but they can affect people who have had diabetes for 15 years or more.

It's important to try to keep your child's blood glucose within a target range, and to set realistic blood glucose goals for children. Tight glucose control—trying to keep glucose levels as close to normal as possible all the time—is usually not recommended for very young children. Young children may have undetected low blood glucose because they are unable to tell someone when they feel symptoms. For example, in a 2-year-old who can't tell you when he feels low, trying to keep his glucose level in the normal range may cause frequent or severe episodes of low blood glucose.

Therefore, blood glucose goals for a child under 6 years of age are generally higher than for older children. Acceptable levels for children under 6 years of age may range from 90–130 mg/dl at fasting and from 90–180 mg/dl at other times.

Developing a treatment plan that meets your child's individual needs, including his eating habits, activity level, and schedule, can help to keep blood glucose levels within the target range. Children and teenagers who do well with their diabetes management seem to follow these practices:

- they eat reasonably, consistently, and on schedule
- they test blood glucose levels frequently
- they adjust insulin frequently

If your child is doing well on his current treatment plan, there may be no need to change anything. But if you and your child are struggling with control issues, you may want to talk with your diabetes health care provider about making changes in the management plan.

THE ROLE OF HEALTH CARE PROVIDERS

One of the lessons of the DCCT was that people who worked with a group of health care providers were more successful at managing their diabetes than people who did not. This group is sometimes called a multi-disciplinary health care team. The advantage of working with a health care team is that you have easy access to several different kinds of help. Health care teams usually work in big hospitals or diabetes centers. Members of the team can include the following people.

- A *doctor* who specializes in diabetes can help you make decisions about what kind of insulin your child should take, what dosage regimen works best for your child, and how to handle sick days. A specialist in diabetes is called a *diabetologist or endocrinologist.*

- A *diabetes educator,* who is often a nurse, can teach you most of the skills you will need to control your child's diabetes and help you learn how to balance food, exercise, and insulin.

- A *dietitian* can teach you about meal planning and nutrition, help you develop a meal plan based on the food preferences of your child, teach you how to handle holidays and parties, and advise you about the special food needs that children with diabetes have.

- A *social worker, psychologist, or psychiatrist* may help you, your child, and your family deal with concerns about living with diabetes.

There are many issues to deal with in the care of children with diabetes. It is often very difficult for the average primary care provider to keep up on new treatment strategies and new technologies. Therefore, if it is possible for you to go to a center that focuses on pediatric diabetes, it would most likely be in your and your child's best interest to do so.

If you live a long way from a health care team, you may need to go to your local family doctor or pediatrician for your child's diabetes care. Sometimes, this doctor might suggest that you go to a diabetes center for an update at least once a year. Or your doctor may be able to refer you to other health care providers in your community who can advise you about meal planning, school schedules, insulin adjustments, and coping with stress. It is most important, however, that someone experienced and knowledgeable about the treatment of childhood diabetes follow your child's health.

KEEPING YOUR CHILD'S BEST INTERESTS AT HEART

The number one player on the health care team is, of course, your child. Your child's physical, mental, and emotional needs are most important. When working with your health care providers (or with other adults in positions of authority, such as teachers at your child's school), you are your child's advocate. You know your child better than anyone. No one else understands his lifestyle, personality, likes, and dislikes as well as you do.

Share what you know about your child openly and honestly with your health care providers, caregivers, and your child's teachers. Your child will benefit from your active participation in decisions about his daily care.

The dietitian included fat-free (skim) milk in 4-year-old Andy's meal plan, but Andy doesn't like milk (especially skim milk). Andy's mother knew he would never drink the milk and that it would be a battle for everyone if he had to drink it. She explained the problem honestly to the dietitian. Having this information enabled the dietitian to change Andy's meal plan, replacing the milk with liquids that Andy liked and would drink. This made it easier for both Andy and his mother to follow the meal plan.

Your child depends on you to support him and to speak on his behalf. Very young children often cannot communicate their needs to adults. Older children may have difficulty expressing their real feelings to adults whom they are taught to respect.

Twelve-year-old Missy knew how to give her own insulin injections, but on school mornings when she was in a hurry she relied on her parents to give her insulin. Missy dreaded going for her diabetes checkups because she thought that the doctor wanted her to be giving all of her own injections all the time. Missy felt the doctor just didn't understand, but she had trouble telling the doctor how she felt. When she told her dad what was bothering her, her dad agreed to talk to the doctor. Together, Missy, her dad, and the doctor agreed on a plan. On school mornings, Missy and her parents would alternate giving her insulin injections. In the evenings and on weekends, Missy would do all of her own injections. This experience taught Missy that open and honest communication works best, that her dad would be her advocate, and that the doctor would negotiate if he understood the problem.

Make sure that the goals set for your child's diabetes care are realistic, both for him and for you. Goals should be agreed on by everyone as both important and achievable.

Fifteen-year-old Joel, who had had diabetes since he was 8, knew he should test his blood glucose four times a day, but he hated doing it. On a good day, he did two blood tests. When Joel wanted to apply for his driver's license, his doctor said that she needed to assess Joel's diabetes control before signing the application. To make the assessment, the doctor needed more blood tests from Joel. Together, Joel, his mother, and the doctor set a goal. Joel would test his blood glucose three or more times a day for one month and record the results. At the end of the month, the three of them would look at the test results to assess Joel's diabetes control. Joel was willing to do this because it took him a step closer to getting something he really wanted—his driver's license.

As a parent, you may need to educate others involved in your child's life. Often those unfamiliar with type 1 diabetes have many misconceptions and misunderstandings about it.

Three-year-old Amanda loved to play with her friends during preschool. After Amanda was diagnosed with diabetes, her mom noticed she was coming home from school quiet and withdrawn. On her volunteer day at the school, Amanda's mom discovered why: Amanda's classmates seemed to be avoiding her and even the teacher kept her distance. Amanda's mom asked to speak with the class the next day and brought in a teddy bear, a juice box, and a bottle of insulin. She explained diabetes to the children, showed them the teddy bear needed juice or insulin to feel better, and stressed that no one could catch diabetes from Amanda. Afterward, Amanda came home from school smiling.

The Nitty-Gritty 1— Insulin Treatment

Everyone who has type 1 diabetes needs insulin injections because there is not enough insulin being made by the body. Insulin must be taken so that it can enter the bloodstream directly, because if insulin is taken by mouth, it is digested like protein and doesn't have any effect on blood glucose levels. Insulin is normally injected into the fatty tissue under the skin. From there, it is absorbed into the bloodstream, then travels to all parts of the body.

WHAT KINDS OF INSULIN ARE THERE?

The first insulin came mostly from cows and pigs. Human insulin, which is made in a laboratory, is now widely available, is less costly to make, and causes fewer allergic reactions than animal insulin. Different kinds of insulin work differently in terms of length of action and peak times (see pages 18–19).

If your child is doing well on her current insulin, there may be no need to change the type of insulin she uses. If not, however, you may want to talk to your doctor about different combinations of insulin doses or how she is getting her insulin (called the delivery system). Insulin can be delivered to the body in many different ways, including syringes, pumps, pens, infusers, and jet injectors. Ask about which delivery system would work best for your child. It isn't a good idea to switch insulin types, brands, or delivery systems without talking to your doctor or diabetes educator about it first.

Insulin allergy is very rare. However, if your child has redness or itching at the needle site, you may need to change the insulin type.

Types of Insulin

Different types of insulin work for different lengths of time in the body. There are rapid-acting, short-acting, intermediate-acting, and long-acting insulins.

■ **Rapid-acting (Humalog or lispro)** insulin begins to work almost immediately after being injected. It works hardest for about an hour after injection and may last from 2–4 hours after injection (this is called the **peak**). This insulin works best to handle high blood glucose after eating, or bring a high blood glucose level down.

■ **Short-acting (regular)** insulin starts to work within half an hour after the injection is given. It works best 2–5 hours after the injection. Regular insulin is usually given 30–45 minutes before a meal.

■ **Intermediate-acting (NPH or lente)** insulin usually works for about 12–18 hours. The peak may be 4–15 hours after the injection. This type of insulin is often given in the morning and evening.

■ **Long-acting (ultralente)** insulin can work for 18–20 hours. It starts to work after 6–10 hours and does not peak. It is injected once or twice a day.

HOW DO I HANDLE INSULIN?

For general storage, it's a good idea to keep bottles of insulin in the refrigerator (in the butter keeper or somewhere else where it will not freeze). Insulin can break down and not work if it gets too cold (less than 36° F) or too warm (over 86° F).

However, you can carry insulin with you in a purse or backpack. Insulin is stable at room temperature as long as it is stored away from heat and light. If your child uses up a bottle of insulin in less than a month, it's okay to keep it at room temperature. If she uses small amounts of insulin, it is generally recommended that you discard the unused portion a month after being opened. It's a good idea to keep the bottle in the carton to protect it from light and keep it clean. Airport X-ray machines do not hurt insulin.

Some people prefer to keep insulin in the refrigerator and take it out for a few minutes to warm up before giving the injection. Others don't seem to notice if the insulin is cool when injected.

HOW MUCH INSULIN DOES MY CHILD NEED?

Insulin dosages are based on your child's height, weight, metabolic rate, physical maturity, activity level, and usual meal plan. A heavier or taller child may need more insulin than a smaller child, and a child who isn't active may need more insulin than one who is.

One 12-year-old may take a total morning dose of 30 units while another 12-year-old takes only 20 units. Taking a larger dose of insulin doesn't mean the child's diabetes is more severe. Different dosages simply mean that children are different, and their bodies have different requirements.

Your child's need for insulin will change from one year to the next, one season to the next, and sometimes one day to the next. This is why it is important to monitor blood glucose frequently so that you can determine your child's insulin needs. Generally, as children grow, they need more insulin. Many children need more insulin in winter than in summer because of differences in their activity level. In winter kids are often less active, are in school, and are indoors more, whereas in the summer they are outside playing all day.

AVAILABLE INSULINS

Many new insulins are being made and tested. Always check to find out which insulins are available since the list is constantly changing.

Product	Manufacturer	Form
Rapid acting (onset < 15 minutes)		
Humalog (lispro)	Lilly	Human
Humalog cartridges	Lilly	Human
Short acting (onset > 30 minutes)		
Humulin R (regular)	Lilly	Human
Humulin R cartridges	Lilly	Human
Iletin II regular	Lilly	Pork
Novolin R (regular)	NovoNordisk	Human
Novolin R Penfill	NovoNordisk	Human
Novolin R Prefilled	NovoNordisk	Human
Velosulin (buffered)	NovoNordisk	Human
Intermediate acting (onset 2–4 hours)		
Humulin L (lente)	Lilly	Human
Humulin N (NPH)	Lilly	Human
Iletin II (lente)	Lilly	Pork
Iletin II (NPH)	Lilly	Pork
Novolin L (lente)	NovoNordisk	Human
Novolin N (NPH)	NovoNordisk	Human
Long acting (onset 6–10 hours)		
Humulin U (ultralente)	Lilly	Human
Mixtures		
Humulin 50/50 (50% NPH, 50% regular)	Lilly	Human
Humulin 70/30 (70% NPH, 30% regular)	Lilly	Human
Humulin 70/30 cartridges	Lilly	Human
Novolin 70/30 (70% NPH, 30% regular)	NovoNordisk	Human
Novolin 70/30 Penfilled	NovoNordisk	Human
Novolin 70/30 Prefilled	NovoNordisk	Human
Novolin 70/25 Penfilled (NPH/lispro)	NovoNordisk	Human

For a few days or months after a child is diagnosed with diabetes, she may need only a very low dose of insulin. During this period, which is sometimes called the "honeymoon period," the child's pancreas still produces some insulin. However, as time goes by, the insulin-producing beta cells are destroyed. As these cells produce less and less insulin, your child will need more insulin by injection.

Big changes in your child's insulin dosage should *only* be made after discussion with your doctor or diabetes educator, but fine-tuning your child's dosage from day to day is something you can and should learn to do yourself (see page 41).

HOW OFTEN DOES MY CHILD NEED INSULIN INJECTIONS?

In the recent past, children with diabetes were given one or two injections of insulin a day. However, after the DCCT showed that multiple daily injections (MDI) worked well for teens and adults, many practitioners have started recommending MDI for children as well. MDI is a form of intensive diabetes management where the aim is to keep blood glucose levels as close to normal as possible all the time. The MDI regimen tries to mimic the way a normal pancreas works, releasing bursts of insulin after each meal and maintaining a 24-hour baseline insulin level to keep the blood glucose stable.

Multiple injections provide a bit more flexibility: the insulin dosage can be adjusted frequently during the day according to food intake and activity level. The same is true for insulin pump therapy, where instead of taking insulin by injection, the pump provides a steady infusion of insulin all the time and is programmed to provide extra insulin to cover food. (For more about pump therapy, see page 34.)

The development of very fine, comfortable needles for injection and the use of rapid-acting insulin makes a MDI regimen more feasible for children. Most children now control diabetes with three or four insulin injections a day. However, some children may be well managed on two injections a day. The number of daily injections your child needs will be based on:

■ the type of insulin your child is taking

- how able and motivated your child is to care for her diabetes herself
- the quality of family and other support available
- your child's level of blood glucose control
- your child's schedule, exercise level, and meal plan
- patterns of blood glucose that emerge with frequent monitoring

Children and teens almost always take more than one kind of insulin. They may take rapid-acting insulin with a meal to balance their intake of food. Before breakfast, before dinner, or at bedtime, they may take an intermediate- or long-acting insulin that works for a longer time.

To avoid gaps or overlaps between doses, a good rule of thumb is to always give the injections at regular times, within about an hour of the usual time. For more on scheduling meals and insulin injections, see the box on the next page.

Rapid-acting (lispro) insulin is usually given immediately before meals or with food. Parents of young children, however, may give it immediately after the meal when they have seen what their child has actually eaten. With this insulin, there should be no waiting period, as it works quickly.

Regular insulin should be given 30 to 45 minutes before a meal. That will give it time to begin to work before the food is digested. The only time when it may not be smart to wait after an injection is if your child is hypoglycemic to start with. If your child's blood glucose is less than 70 mg/dl, or she has symptoms of hypoglycemia, you should feed your child and then inject the insulin.

NPH, lente, or ultralente insulin should be given at the usual times, but there is no requirement about waiting to eat, since their purpose is to provide a long-term baseline insulin level, rather than to help with any particular meal.

During summer vacation and at other times when your child's schedule changes, it's okay to gradually alter the times of insulin injections. For example, if your child wants to get up and eat breakfast later during the summer months, the whole schedule

SCHEDULING MEALS AND INSULIN INJECTIONS

A helpful rule of thumb is to give injections and have meals about the same time, give or take an hour. Here's how this might work.

Usual getting-up time: 7 a.m.

■ Give the injection of intermediate-acting insulin no earlier than 6 a.m. and no later than 8 a.m.

Usual breakfast time: 7:30 a.m.

■ Eat breakfast no earlier than 6:30 a.m. and no later than 8:30 a.m. If your child takes short-acting (regular) insulin, give the injection 30 minutes before breakfast, if possible, or use a regular/NPH mixture. If your child takes rapid-acting (lispro) insulin, give the injection immediately before eating.

Usual lunch time: noon

■ Eat lunch no earlier than 11 a.m. and no later than 1 p.m. If your child takes short-acting (regular) insulin, give the injection 30 minutes before lunch, if possible. If your child takes rapid-acting (lispro) insulin, give the injection immediately before eating.

Usual dinner time: 5 p.m.

■ Eat dinner no earlier than 4 p.m. and no later than 6 p.m. Give the injection of intermediate-acting insulin no earlier than 4 p.m. and no later than 6 p.m. If your child takes short-acting (regular) insulin, give the injection 30 minutes before dinner, if possible. If your child takes rapid-acting (lispro) insulin, give the injection immediately before eating.

can be pushed back. Your doctor or diabetes educator can help you decide how to handle these kinds of schedule changes.

GIVING THE INJECTIONS

Giving your child an insulin injection can be hard, both emotionally and physically, especially if your child is young and squirms a lot. The material presented here may give you some guidance.

HOW TO DRAW UP ONE TYPE OF INSULIN

1. Wash your hands.
2. Select the injection site according to your rotation schedule (see *What Is Site Rotation?* on page 28).
3. Clean the injection site with soap and water or alcohol. (Alcohol may be used if it is more convenient, but it dries the skin.)

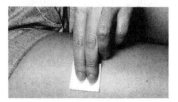

4. If you are using NPH, lente, or ultralente, gently roll the insulin bottle between your hands to mix the insulin. Wipe the top of the insulin bottle with alcohol.

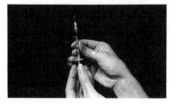

5. Draw back the plunger on the syringe to the correct number of insulin units.

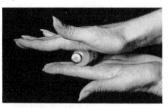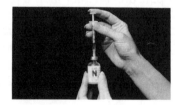

6. Holding the insulin bottle upright, insert the needle into the bottle and push the plunger in. This injects air into the bottle.

(*continued*)

How to Draw Up One Type of Insulin *(continued)*

7. Keeping the needle in the bottle, turn the bottle upside down and slowly pull back the plunger until the syringe has more insulin in it than you need.

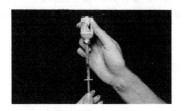

8. Gently tap the syringe to move air bubbles to the top.
9. With the needle still in the bottle, slowly press the plunger forward to expel the air bubbles and extra insulin.

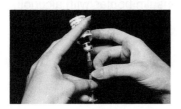

10. Double-check that you have the correct number of insulin units in the syringe.

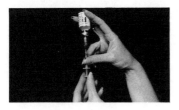

11. Gently pull the needle out of the bottle.

If you are using the longer 5/8 mm syringes, gently pinch up the skin in the area where you are giving the injection with one hand. This avoids injecting the insulin into a muscle, which can be painful and can also alter the way insulin is absorbed by the body.

HOW TO DRAW UP TWO TYPES OF INSULIN

1. Wash your hands thoroughly.
2. Select the injection site according to your rotation schedule (see *What Is Site Rotation?* on page 28).
3. Clean the injection site with soap and water or alcohol. (Alcohol may be used if it is more convenient, but it dries the skin.)

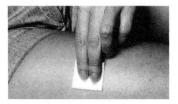

4. Gently roll the cloudy insulin bottle between your hands to mix the insulin. Wipe the top of the insulin bottles with alcohol.

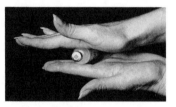

5. Draw back the plunger on the syringe to the correct number of units of rapid- or short-acting (clear) insulin to be given.

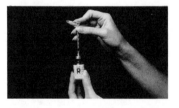

6. Holding the bottle of short-acting insulin upright, insert the needle into the air space in the bottle and push the plunger in. This injects air into the bottle. Remove the needle.

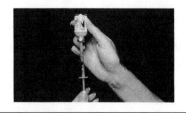

How to Draw Up Two Types of Insulin (*continued*)

7. Draw back the plunger on the syringe to the correct number of units of intermediate-acting (cloudy) insulin to be given.
8. Holding the bottle of intermediate-acting insulin upright, insert the needle into the bottle and push the plunger in. This injects air into the bottle.
9. Keeping the needle in the bottle, turn the bottle of intermediate-acting insulin upside down and slowly pull back the plunger until the syringe has more insulin in it than you need.
10. Gently tap the syringe to move air bubbles to the top.

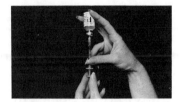

11. With the needle still in the bottle, slowly press the plunger forward to expel the air bubbles and extra insulin.
12. Double-check that you have the correct number of units of intermediate-acting insulin in the syringe.
13. Gently pull the needle out of the bottle of intermediate-acting insulin.
14. Insert the needle into the bottle of short-acting insulin and slowly withdraw the correct number of units. *Take care that none of the intermediate-acting insulin already in the syringe is pushed into the bottle of short-acting insulin. If the insulins are accidentally mixed in the bottle, you must discard the bottle of short-acting insulin because it may not act quickly anymore.*
15. Check for air bubbles in the syringe. If there is a large air bubble in the syringe after you have added the short-acting insulin, discard the syringe and start again. If there is a small air bubble that can be tapped out without noticeably changing the dosage, go ahead and give the injection. Small air bubbles will not harm your child, but they can alter the amount of insulin injected.

The advantage of drawing up the intermediate-acting (cloudy) insulin first and then the short-acting (clear) insulin is that you can see your mistake immediately if you accidentally push cloudy insulin into the bottle of clear insulin. Another way of doing it would be to draw up the short-acting (clear) insulin first. This lessens the risk of contaminating the bottle of short-acting insulin.

HOW TO GIVE AN INSULIN INJECTION

■ If you are using the short needle syringes, hold the syringe like a pencil and insert the needle gently at a 90° angle to the skin (straight up and down).

■ Push gently but steadily on the plunger.

■ Give the injection quickly or slowly, depending on your child's preference.

■ Pull the needle out and throw it immediately (uncapped) into a proper disposal container (a "sharps box").

■ After the injection, praise your child for doing a good job and give her a big hug.

With the newer short needle syringes, it is not necessary to pinch up the skin. In the overweight child, these needles may not be deep enough to allow adequate absorption. Some children report that the short syringes hurt more, possibly because the depth of penetration is closer to nerves on the surface.

WHAT IS SITE ROTATION?

Giving your child's insulin injections in different places is called site rotation. Rotating insulin injection sites is important so that puffy, lumpy spots do not develop and hinder the absorption of insulin. When insulin is injected in the same site over time, it can attract fat into the injection area, leading to the formation of lumps made of fat and scar tissue. Absorption of insulin from the lumps is poor. Injecting into these lumps (or into scar tissue) can slow down insulin action. If insulin is poorly absorbed, your child may have wide swings in blood glucose levels.

The important thing is not how you rotate sites, but that you *do* rotate sites. Every parent and child seems to work out their system a bit differently depending on the child's preferred sites, musculature, and tolerance of injections. Rotating injections according to a plan also helps you and your child remember where the right place is for the injection each time. Being consistent is important.

WHERE TO GIVE INSULIN INJECTIONS

Where to give injections in your child's arm:

▮ Ask your child to put her left hand on her right arm (by the shoulder) with her fingers closed (Figure A). The bottom of the hand is the highest point where injections should be given.

▮ Next, ask your child to grab her arm just above the right elbow (Figure B). The top of the hand is the lowest point where injections should be given.

▮ In the space between your child's hands, draw two imaginary lines down the arm—one down the side and one down the middle of the back of the arm.

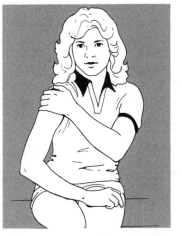

Figure A

▮ Give the injections along these two tracks, measuring from one spot to the next by the width of two of your child's fingers.

Where to give injections in your child's thigh:

▮ Ask your child to put one hand at the top of her thigh (by the hip) and the other hand on top of her knee on the same leg (Figure C). It's okay to give injections in the space between the hands.

▮ Draw three imaginary lines, one down the top of the leg and one on each side—one toward the outside and one toward the inside.

▮ Give the injections along these three tracks, measuring from one spot to the next by the width of two of your child's fingers.

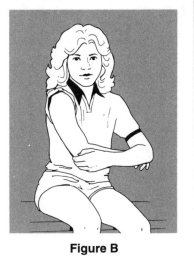

Figure B

Where to Give Insulin Injections *(continued)*

Where to give injections in your child's abdomen:

■ Draw an imaginary one-inch circle around your child's navel.
Don't give injections inside the
circle because this area can be
tender.

■ Give the injections in the sur-
rounding area of the abdomen,
stomach, and hip.

Where to give injections in your child's hip:

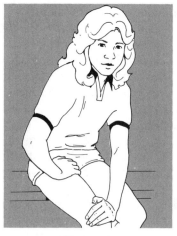

■ The upper outer quadrant of
the buttock (actually the hip) is
a suitable place for injections,
although it may be a difficult
area for your child to reach to
give her own injections. Check

Figure C

with your child's doctor for instructions on giving injections in
the hip (Figure D).

If your child gets puffiness or lumps near the area of an injection:

■ Don't give any more injections
in that spot for 3–6 months.
The lumps should go away.

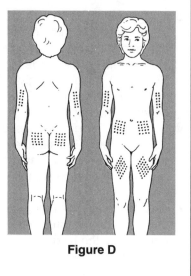

Figure D

Insulin is absorbed most quickly when the injection is given in the abdomen. It is absorbed a bit more slowly when the injection is given in the arms, more slowly still in the legs, and slowest of all when the injection is given in the hip.

Having a plan for rotating where you give your child's injections can help to make sure that insulin is absorbed at the same rate. For example, if your child gets three injections a day, you could give the morning injection in the abdomen, dinner injection in the arm, and the evening injection in the hip.

You may also want to rotate within one area—like the fleshy part of the upper arm—by dividing it with imaginary lines (see page 29).

TIPS FOR EASIER INSULIN INJECTIONS— PART I

If you are worried that the injection hurts your child:

■ Poke yourself in the abdomen with a syringe (but do *not* inject air) to see what the needle feels like. (Or get someone— perhaps your child—to give you the poke.) You may be relieved to find that it hardly hurts at all because the needle is so fine.

If your child wants to give her own injection in the arm:

■ Have her press her arm against a chair or a wall or over a bent knee to help to make the fleshy part of the arm stand out.

If insulin frequently leaks out after you give the injection:

■ Try pulling the skin to one side when pinching it up. When you finish giving the injection and release the skin, it will cover up the needle mark and prevent leaking.
■ After pushing in the plunger, count slowly to 10 before removing the needle.

If the plunger won't push in easily:

■ Pull back slightly on the needle. If the plunger still won't move easily, take the needle out and try giving the injection at another spot.
■ If the plunger still won't move, fill a new syringe and start over. The insulin may be jamming the needle.

TIPS FOR EASIER INSULIN INJECTIONS—
PART II

If your child gets bruising around the area of the injection:

■ Bruising is usually caused by a small broken blood vessel. It's hard to avoid bruising once in awhile. Unless it happens a lot, it isn't something you should worry about. If it does happen a lot, check to see whether it's happening at all injection sites or mostly at one site (such as the arms). Ask your nurse educator for help with your injection technique.

If the area of the injection turns red:

■ Redness may be caused by alcohol that is used to clean the skin. If you use alcohol, allow it to dry thoroughly before giving the injection. If alcohol irritates your child's skin, use soap and water instead.

■ Rarely, redness may be caused by an allergic reaction to insulin. (If your child is taking human insulin, allergic reactions are *extremely* rare.) The spot may be tender or itchy. If your child's injection sites turn red or itchy, tell your doctor about it.

If the injection is painful:

■ An injection may be more painful than usual if:
  ● it is given in dense muscle tissue
  ● it caused a bruise
  ● the injection was given close to a nerve ending
  ● the needle is accidentally blunted when the insulin is withdrawn from the bottle
  ● the needle is inserted too slowly as it goes through the skin
Consult your doctor or diabetes educator if your child frequently complains of pain during injections. However, many children complain more at the idea of having the injection than because the injection is actually painful.

■ An injection aid (injector) may help. Injectors can make it easier to put the needle through the skin or to give injections in hard-to-reach places. This category includes devices that make giving an injection easier (insertion aids), as well as syringe alternatives, including:
  ● infusers (a needle is inserted, usually into the abdomen, and remains taped in place for 48–72 hours)
  ● jet injectors (a tiny stream of insulin is forced through the skin with pressure instead of a puncture)
  ● insulin pens (more on these below)
Your doctor or diabetes educator can give you more information about injection aids.

If your child is having wide swings in blood glucose levels, keeping track of where you give the injections can help you to see if the swings have a pattern that is related to the injection site. (For example, do your child's blood glucose levels swing more when the injections are given in the hip than when they are given in the arms?) Your doctor or diabetes educator can help you and your child decide on the best way to do site rotation.

INSULIN DELIVERY DEVICES

As technology has progressed and multiple daily injections have become more common, the use of insulin pens and insulin pumps has become more popular.

Insulin Pens

The insulin pen has insulin or an insulin cartridge in a device that looks like a pen and is easy to use. People using insulin pens don't have to carry insulin bottles and syringes. Instead, they simply and discreetly pull out the pen and inject as needed. There are disposable needles, however, that must be changed with each injection. The pens are available from manufacturers in several different types of insulin. Some of the pens have a disposable insulin cartridge that is changed when empty, and other pens are completely disposable.

Not every type of insulin is available for insulin pen use. Also, you cannot mix types of insulin together in a special ratio. The pens do come already premixed in standard ratios (70/30 NPH/regular, for example), but the dose cannot be changed as needed, which most children might require. In most cases, children and teens will use the pen to take regular or lispro insulin either before lunch or dinner or both. It is portable, manageable, and the "dial-a-dose" format is easy for kids to do accurately. With the disposable pens, it is now possible for kids to leave one pen at their friend's house, one at Grandma's, and carry one for spontaneous use at a restaurant!

Insulin Pumps

Insulin pump therapy is growing in popularity as an option for the treatment of type 1 diabetes. The insulin pump is a small battery-run device that gives a continuous infusion of insulin through a flexible needle. The soft, comfortable needle is inserted into the abdomen or hip and left in place for 2 days. The pump itself is about the size of a pager and stores a supply of either regular or lispro insulin. It is worn all of the time, but can be disconnected for bathing, swimming, or contact sports. Generally, however, it should not be disconnected for more than an hour at a time.

Using an insulin pump is a form of intensive diabetes management, where the aim is to keep blood glucose levels as close to normal as possible all the time. The idea of pump therapy is to provide flexibility so that you can respond to changes in blood glucose levels, exercise, or food eaten.

Although pump therapy does promote flexibility and convenience, it still takes time, attention, and energy. Pump users must test their blood glucose at least four times a day and be diligent about problem solving. At least at first, it is essential to work closely with a doctor or nurse to decide on insulin dosages or handle any problems that come up.

Although pump therapy is generally safe, and there are alarms on the pump if anything should go wrong, it is easy to develop hyperglycemia if there is a leak or obstruction in the tubing or needle. Because there is no intermediate-acting insulin present, if there is a leak or the needle comes out, it does not take long for high blood glucose and ketones to develop. Therefore, the pump user must be careful about monitoring and be prepared to change the needle site if unexplained high blood glucose should occur. It is also possible to develop infections at the needle site, although this is unusual if good hygiene practices are followed.

Is a Pump Right for My Child?

The use of insulin pump therapy in children is now becoming more widely accepted. However, many children are not developmentally able to handle the responsibility or balk at the idea of having hardware connected to them constantly. Some very young children are now using pumps, especially in some of the major diabetes centers where there is a lot of experienced staff to provide the necessary guidance. School-agers and teens often find the pump useful in responding to changing activity, food, and hormone levels.

Using a pump may be an option for a child or teenager who:

▪ wants a more flexible meal plan or freedom from multiple insulin injections

▪ is mature enough to look after the pump and check her blood glucose levels regularly

▪ recognizes the signs and symptoms of low blood glucose and knows how to treat them when they occur

For a teen who is mostly responsible for her own decisions, a pump can work very well, if she is motivated to care for her diabetes. For a child, however, the burden of responsibility for diabetes care usually falls on the parent, who cannot always be with the child to supervise decisions.

If you and your child are interested in using an insulin pump, you should arrange to see a doctor and a diabetes educator who have experience looking after people who use pumps.

HOW CAN I HELP MY CHILD TO ACCEPT INSULIN INJECTIONS?

Every child is different. Some children adjust well to insulin injections, while others find them very hard to accept. There are several reasons why a child may protest or fight injections.

▪ The injection may be painful or there may be past associations of pain with shots.

- The child may be expressing anger about having diabetes.
- The child may be afraid of needles.
- It may be an age-related problem. For example, preschool children generally do not do well with any kind of intrusive procedure.

You may find it helpful to use an injection aid (see box, page 132). Going over how to give injections with your diabetes educator may also help.

Very young children may fuss during injections. It may help to tell your child that the injection keeps her healthy and to give her a big hug when it's over. The fuss usually subsides over time as your child becomes used to getting injections regularly.

To get your child used to the idea of getting insulin injections, it may help in the beginning to associate the injection with something the child enjoys, like watching a favorite show on television. Say, "Every day, just before you watch XYZ show, Mom (or Dad) will give you an injection to keep you well."

In families where both parents are available, it's a good idea for both to be involved in giving the child's insulin injections. That way, both parents share the responsibility and one parent does not always feel like the bad guy. Also, try to avoid the word "shot." Although commonly used, this word can mean shot with a gun or arrow to children.

It's normal for children to protest about injections at times, especially when they are tired, stressed, or unhappy. However, if your family's life is consistently disrupted by your child's resistance to injections, a social worker or psychologist may be able to help with a plan to smooth things out (see *Asking for Help*, page 140).

WHEN IS MY CHILD READY TO GIVE HER OWN INJECTIONS?

Learning to give their own injections is an important step for children with diabetes because it helps them be more independent. They can go to visit relatives or on sleepovers with friends. Most important, they can feel in charge of their diabetes and not the other way around.

There is no strict rule about when children are ready to start giving their own injections. One child may be ready to do it (with a parent watching) at age 7, while another child may not be ready until age 12. The right age for your child is whenever she is capable of doing it and when both you and the child feel comfortable about her doing it.

Try to be patient and let your child do the injections when she feels ready, but remind her that you are always there to help. She may quickly get the hang of giving her own injections and may do it without your help at all for a while. Then, for some reason, she may again want you to help or to give the injection. It is common for children to move forward and then step back. Sometimes they need reassurance that they can still rely on their parents' support.

Your child may feel okay about giving injections in the legs but not in the arms or abdomen. You may need to keep doing those injections for a while. Or you may want to suggest that you give

ENCOURAGING YOUR CHILD TO GIVE HER OWN INJECTIONS

Encourage your child a step at a time to take responsibility for giving her own insulin injections.

- Start by asking your child to choose the injection site, to clean the site, or to prepare the dose.
- Then suggest that your child push in the plunger or take the needle out of the skin after the injection.
- As your child becomes more comfortable doing these things, suggest that she hold the syringe.
- Give your child lots of praise as she takes on greater responsibility for injections.
- Eventually, your child will be able to do the whole procedure herself!

the injections on odd-numbered days and that your child gives them on even-numbered days.

Wanting to go on a camping trip or sleepover at a friend's house may give your child an incentive to learn to do her own injections. Getting to know other children who can give their own injections may also help. Encourage your child to attend a youth group or a camp for children with diabetes. And don't be surprised if a letter home from camp announces with pride, "I gave my own injection today!" (See *Should I Send My Child to Diabetes Camp?* on page 116.)

Even when you feel comfortable about your child giving her own injections, supervision is recommended. A responsible adult should check to make sure the dose is correct and that all the insulin is injected. Children (even teenagers) always feel more secure when their parents are involved in their diabetes care.

HOW DO WE DISPOSE OF NEEDLES?

It's important to handle and dispose of used needles and lancets safely. It's safest to not recap needles or lancets. This helps you avoid being accidentally stuck. Your diabetes educator may be able to get you a special box to use for disposing of needles and lancets (called a "sharps box"). Otherwise, use a plastic milk carton or a soda or detergent bottle. Check with your local trash disposal company to find out how to label and dispose of the used needle container.

ADJUSTING INSULIN AT HOME

Your child's insulin doses may vary from day to day. With help from your health care provider, you will learn how to make small adjustments in your child's daily insulin dosage depending on what she has to eat and how active she is. Major changes in your child's insulin dose should only be made with the guidance of your doctor or diabetes educator. However, you can make small (within 10% of the usual dose) changes yourself.

Fine-tuning your child's dosage helps to keep her blood glucose levels in the target range. Looking for patterns in glucose levels will help you to adjust the insulin dose. The point of making small adjustments frequently is to prevent both high and low blood glucose. Sometimes you may make adjustments and they don't seem to be working, but try to think how it might be if you didn't try at all. Sometimes discussing your changes with your health care provider will give you some insight into the problem.

Remember, too, that neither the amount of insulin nor the number of injections your child needs is a measure of the severity of her diabetes. As your child grows, she will need more insulin. Growth hormone, and all of the hormones of puberty, cause insulin needs to go higher. If there is not enough insulin present, her growth may not reach its full potential. As your child grows and needs more insulin, it doesn't mean her diabetes has gotten worse—she's gotten bigger!

How Do Food and Exercise Affect My Child's Insulin Needs?

The amount of insulin your child needs from day to day is affected by how much and what type of food she eats and how active she is. Your diabetes educator can help you learn how to make daily adjustments to your child's insulin dosage depending on the food and activities planned for that day.

Food raises blood glucose while exercise lowers it. Eating more than usual or eating a sugar-rich food like birthday cake can make your child's blood glucose rise. Taking part in a strenuous game can make it drop.

Extra food helps to balance exercise. When your child is going to exercise, you can decrease insulin, give her more food to eat, or both. When blood glucose runs high, you can give more insulin

Stacey is on the high school swim team. She has swim practice every day at 3 p.m. She has a snack before practice, but she doesn't want to eat a lot of food right before swimming. However, she also doesn't want to start feeling low while she's in the pool. In the morning, Stacey takes intermediate-acting (NPH) insulin every morning which is working at peak effectiveness at about 3 p.m. To prevent a low during swim practice, Stacey reduces her NPH dose by 2 units.

or adjust the child's meal plan so she is eating less. If your child is going through a phase when she is eating less than usual, she will need less insulin. Your doctor or diabetes educator can help you to understand how to balance food, activity, and insulin to keep your child's blood glucose level in the target range. (See *Playing Games and Sports Safely*, page 72, and *The Nitty-Gritty 3— Meal Planning*, page 53, for more on how food and exercise affect your child's need for insulin.)

James, who is 11 years old, is going on an overnight scout camping trip. When James is camping, his glucose levels are usually in his target range because of all the games and activities. But the troop is planning to roast marshmallows and make popcorn at the campfire. James wants to eat the marshmallows with his friends, but they will probably raise his blood glucose.

His mom suggests that he test his blood glucose before the campfire. She tells him that his blood sugar will probably be okay from all of the games played that evening. She writes the following note for James:

Dear James,

Enjoy 4 to 6 cups of popcorn! And . . . .
Eat 6 marshmallows if your blood test is less than 80.
Eat 4 marshmallows if your blood test is 80 to 180.
Eat 2 marshmallows if your blood test is over 180.

Love, Mom

How Do I Fine-Tune My Child's Dosage?

Fine-tuning your child's insulin dosage means:

- learning to look for patterns of high or low blood glucose
- trying to figure out why high or low blood glucose levels occur
- adjusting your child's insulin dose, food, or timing of meals to fix the problem

If your child's blood glucose level is a bit too high, you can increase the insulin dose or reduce food. If your child's blood glucose level is a bit too low, you can decrease the dose or add food. When glucose is:

High ↑ Increase insulin

Low ↓ Decrease insulin

However, there are some exceptions to this rule (see *Rebound (Somogyi Effect)*, page 86).

The box below gives an example of how insulin doses can be adjusted according to blood glucose level. Your doctor or diabetes

---

ADJUSTMENT SCALE FOR REGULAR OR LISPRO INSULIN

Find the blood glucose range in the column on the left. Then look at the column on the right to find the corresponding insulin dose. For example, if Jimmy's blood glucose reading is 142 mg/dl, he should take 5 units of insulin.

Subtract 2 units if your child will be exercising strenuously. For example, if Jimmy's blood glucose reading is 135 mg/dl but he will be playing soccer after breakfast, he should take 3 units of insulin.

Blood glucose reading (mg/dl) (before breakfast)	Insulin dose
<70	3 units
70–120	4 units
121–180	5 units
181–240	6 units
241–300	7 units
>301	8 units

educator can prepare a dosage adjustment chart or scale that's right for your child.

Why Are Patterns in Blood Glucose Levels Important?

It may take a few days for a dosage adjustment to make a difference in your child's blood glucose control. So it is important to look for patterns in blood glucose levels over periods of three or four days.

Like most children, your child probably takes more than one type of insulin. For example, she may take a mixture of intermediate-acting (NPH) and rapid-acting (lispro) insulin in the morning, lispro insulin before dinner, and NPH before her bedtime snack. This means that at different times of day a different type of insulin is working in your child's body.

> Mike had soccer practice from 7 to 8 p.m. on Mondays, Wednesdays, and Fridays. Halfway through practice he would have symptoms of hypoglycemia. To prevent low blood glucose during soccer practice, Mike reduced his before-dinner dose of lispro insulin by 2 units on soccer nights.

Knowing what is causing a problem, as well as what time of day a problem is occurring, can help you decide how to fine-tune your child's dosage. This is why blood glucose testing throughout the day is so important.

The Nitty-Gritty 2—Glucose Testing

Regular testing of blood glucose levels is a very important part of your child's diabetes care. It's the only way to know if your child's blood glucose level is in the target range. If your child has many blood glucose readings outside of the target range you may need to change her insulin dose, food, or schedule.

Glucose testing means using a meter to measure the amount of glucose in a drop of capillary blood, usually from a finger. Glucose meters are so easy to use that most children can quickly learn how to do their own glucose tests.

Knowing your child's blood glucose level before a meal can help you to decide whether to encourage him to eat an extra helping of food or to give more or less than the usual insulin dose at the next injection.

Learning to look for patterns in your child's blood glucose levels will help you to fine-tune his insulin dosages, activity level, and food intake. Your doctor or diabetes educator can help you to do this.

HOW OFTEN SHOULD MY CHILD'S BLOOD GLUCOSE BE TESTED?

How often your child's blood glucose level needs to be tested depends on your child's needs. His age, eating habits, activity level, and insulin needs, as well as how quickly he is growing, all need to be considered in determining how frequently blood should be tested.

At a minimum, four blood glucose tests a day are usually recommended for children and teens. Testing blood glucose levels during the night also gives helpful information about how to regulate food and insulin and can help detect nighttime low blood glucose. Children on multiple daily injections or an insulin pump will need to test at least four times a day. The more tests that are done, the more information is available to keep blood glucose in the target range.

Frequent blood glucose tests are especially important in very young children who can't talk because they can't tell you whether they are feeling symptoms of low or high blood glucose. *When in doubt—test!*

Other Times to Do Blood Glucose Tests

Your doctor may sometimes ask you to test your child's blood glucose levels at other times of day than when you usually do it. This can help you to get a clearer picture of what happens to your child's glucose levels throughout the day.

DOING THE FINGERSTICK

1. Wash your child's hands with warm, soapy water and dry well.
2. Prepare your meter and test strip according to the manufacturer's instructions.
3. Choose the spot where you are going to do the fingerstick.
4. Place the finger-pricking device on the side of the finger. Press the release mechanism.
5. Squeeze out a drop of blood. If you have a hard time drawing a drop of blood, try this:
   - after sticking the finger, hang the hand down and gently shake it
   - lightly squeeze the finger, moving from the middle joint toward the fingertip (this is called "milking" the finger)
6. Place the blood as directed in the instructions for your meter.
7. Wait for the results. Record the number in your daily log.

TIPS FOR EASIER, LESS PAINFUL STICKS

▌ New pricking devices and fine pointed lancets help to make the stick almost painless. Some of these devices are specially made for children's sensitive fingers. They go deep enough into the skin to draw a small drop of blood but not deep enough to hurt much or leave much of a mark. Ask your diabetes educator or pharmacist to show you these devices.

▌ Prick the sides of the fingers to draw blood. The sides have a good blood supply and fewer nerve endings than the fingertips.

▌ In young children with tiny fingers, you can also do sticks in the earlobes, heels, and toes. (In infants, it is safest to use the outer sides of the heels.)

For example, your child's blood glucose may always be normal before meals. But how do you know whether it goes sky high right after meals? The way to find out is to sometimes do a test an hour or two after a meal. You can use the additional information you get from these tests to help you make decisions about your child's daily food intake and his exercise and insulin routine.

It can also be helpful to check blood glucose after your child eats a food that you suspect raises his glucose level unusually high. This can help you to decide whether to give extra insulin before your child eats that food next time. Extra blood tests when your child is sick can help you decide how to adjust insulin dosages and food. Anytime that your child acts like or says he feels his blood glucose is low, it's a good idea to do a blood test. This can prevent anxious eating, when a child mistakes nervousness for low blood glucose and eats a snack he doesn't need.

Checking blood glucose is helpful before, during, and after exercise. If your child's blood glucose is on the low side before exercise, you can see that he eats an extra snack. Doing a check during exercise can show you if your child's sweating and pounding heart are caused by exertion or by low blood glucose. (See *Playing Games and Sports Safely*, page 72.)

Your doctor or diabetes educator will help you to look for patterns in your child's blood glucose readings and decide whether your child's insulin dose needs to be changed.

RECORDING RESULTS OF BLOOD GLUCOSE TESTS

Each time you do a blood glucose test, it's very important to record the reading. A log will help you to keep track of this information.

Most meters have a memory that holds a variable number of previous readings. Some meters include the date and time of the test and can be downloaded into a computer program. This is helpful if you forget to record the blood glucose results. But if you rely on the memory and don't keep records of insulin and events, not only can you miss patterns of control, but you won't know the reasons for anything unusual.

Some of the newer meters have the ability to record events such as a sweet food eaten or extra exercise done. You need to be diligent about putting this information into your meter, if you are not using a hand-written log. The records are your tools for improving diabetes control.

Look at your records frequently. After downloading your meter into the computer, some people find it helpful to sort their information into graphs and charts. Most logs have a comments section for recording events during the day, such as exercise, meal times, special treats eaten, low blood glucose symptoms, or illness. These records can help you detect patterns and trends in glucose levels. There is a sample log on page 48.

HOW DO I KNOW IF I'M TESTING BLOOD GLUCOSE CORRECTLY?

Remember to take your meter and your log of written records with you when you go to see your health care provider. He or she may want to check the meter to make sure it is working accurately.

Blood glucose meters are now making blood glucose testing very easy to do. Most meters are accurate and designed to be simple to use. Your health care provider can teach you how to do blood glucose testing correctly and answer any questions that you may have. In addition, the manufacturers of meters always have customer service departments that you can call with questions or concerns.

MAKING SURE YOUR METER IS ACCURATE

Every brand of meter allows you to check its accuracy so that you know your results are true. This is done in a variety of ways. One way is to use a control solution. Control solutions are made to work with the brand of meter they are sold for, so be sure not to cross brands. The results you get with the check strip or control solution should be within a certain range. If after testing you find that your meter is out of the accepted range for accuracy, call the customer service phone number for your brand of meter.

Another way of checking the accuracy of your meter is to compare a sample of blood on your meter with a laboratory result for the blood. This works best when the same sample of blood is used for both. This needs to be done when you visit your health care provider, because you will use blood taken from a vein rather than from the capillaries in the finger. Glucose results from capillary blood are about 11% higher than with blood from a vein. If the reading from your meter and the result from the laboratory are within 20% of each other, your meter is accurate. You should also know whether your meter is scaled to blood serum or whole blood. Serum values are higher.

URINE TESTING

Urine can be tested for the presence of glucose and/or the presence of ketones.

Diabetes Weekly Diary

Insulin (Brand, Type, Species)

Month: **Year:**

Date/Day	Insulin Dose					Blood Glucose and Urine Ketone Test Results							
	Time / Units					Breakfast		Lunch	Dinner	Bedtime	Night	Comments/Exercise/Injection Sites
						Urine	Blood	Blood	Blood	Blood		

Urine testing can be a useful way to tell if blood glucose levels have been high, especially overnight. If your child's blood glucose level is normal in the morning but there is a lot of glucose in his urine, it's likely that his glucose level ran high sometime during the night. However, urine glucose testing is not a substitute for blood glucose testing.

Most importantly, urine testing checks for *ketones*. Ketones are by-products of breaking down body fat. The body breaks down fat for energy when glucose is not reaching cells. Ketones can appear in the urine when your child has:

- an illness
- not taken enough insulin
- emotional stress
- not been eating well
- recently had an episode of low blood glucose

Report the presence of ketones in the urine to your medical team, and together you can figure out what's going on.

When your child is sick, test for ketones every time he urinates. Tell your doctor or nurse if you find a large amount of ketones in your child's urine or if ketones are present (even in small amounts) on more than one test.

Ketones can cause the blood to become acidic, which leads to nausea, vomiting, and flu-like symptoms. Large amounts of

---

CHECKING GLUCOSE LEVELS IN URINE

There are several methods of testing for glucose in urine. Follow the directions that come with the test strip. A negative reading means there is no glucose in the urine. A reading of 5 percent means there are 5 grams of glucose per deciliter (or 50 grams in 1 liter) of urine.

A high urine glucose means that the blood glucose level has been above 180 mg/dl at some point since the child last urinated.

ketones in the urine can lead to a dangerous condition called ketoacidosis. (See page 85.)

Ask your doctor for more specific guidance on whom to call and what to do when you find ketones in your child's urine.

HELPING YOUR CHILD TEST REGULARLY

Getting your child to do blood glucose testing four or more times a day can be a challenge. Your child may resist testing because he does not feel it is important or doesn't want to get bad news. Sometimes children will say they didn't test because they "knew" they were either high or low. (Research has shown that children and adults cannot accurately guess their blood glucose much of the time.) At times your child may find it hard to do the testing himself, and you may have to take over for a while.

Giving praise each time a test is done or awarding stars or points toward an extra privilege or special fun event can help to get your young child to test regularly. In time, the need for these kinds of motivators usually fades away, but continual positive reinforcement remains important. Let your child know that even high numbers give the information needed to control blood glucose.

WHAT IS THE GLYCATED HEMOGLOBIN (HbA$_{1c}$) TEST?

The HbA$_{1c}$ test is a useful blood test that your doctor should do to measure your child's average blood glucose control over a period of a couple of months.

Chris thought that doing his blood tests took too much time. He had more homework now that he was in high school. On top of this, he had basketball practices and a part-time job. Chris' parents also quizzed him about everything he ate if his glucose reading was high. Chris found that it was easier to just write in some glucose values in his log rather than actually doing the test. Plus, he could write glucose readings that were within his target range and get his parents off his case.

When he had his diabetes appointment, the diabetes educator checked his meter's memory and learned that the glucose values didn't match with his log book. Chris was afraid that his parents and doctor would be angry with him. He was glad that instead of showing disappointment, the doctor and his parents made a deal with him.

The nurse worked with Chris and found out which times of the day he could test without it being a hassle. Chris, his parents, the nurse, and the doctor agreed to a testing schedule that would really work. His parents agreed not to pressure him when he missed a test or if his readings were high. Chris promised to record glucose readings that were real. If Chris successfully worked within the agreement, his parents would allow him to get his driver's permit.

The test measures glycated hemoglobin (HbA_1 or HbA_{1c}). Hemoglobin is a substance in red blood cells. HbA is a type of hemoglobin to which glucose attaches. If your child's blood glucose is high, the level of HbA will be high as well. Because the results of the HbA_{1c} test are not affected by last-minute efforts at control, the test acts as a check on average blood glucose control over a several-month period. This is one of the ways that clinicians determine how well a child's blood glucose level is controlled.

It is important to keep in mind that anything that causes a high blood glucose level, such as illness or stress, can affect the HbA_{1c} value. For example, strep throat caused your child's blood glucose levels to be high, so his HbA_{1c} result is affected. Sometimes life gets in the way of the best control, so if it happens that your child's test result is higher than you would like it to be, use this number as a new starting point and work toward an improvement for the next time.

The HbA_{1c} test was one of the tools used in the Diabetes Control and Complications Trial (see page 11). One of the things doctors tried to do in this study was to get patients' HbA_{1c} levels as close to normal as possible. This can be hard to do, especially in children and teenagers. But we now know that keeping HbA_{1c} levels close to normal may help to delay or prevent complications of diabetes. (See *Complications of Diabetes*, page 94.)

The HbA_{1c} test is considered to be a very important part of diabetes care. Make sure that your child is having this test done at least every three months and that the results are given to you. There are now home tests for HbA_{1c} available. Use these results to guide your adjustments and management.

Sam's blood glucose test records indicated that his glucose level was in the target range most of the time, but his HbA_{1c} test results were high. This told the doctor that Sam may not be testing at the times his blood glucose readings are high, or that there could be a problem with the way Sam or his parents are doing blood glucose testing or recording test results.

The Nitty-Gritty 3—
Meal Planning

Food is a very important part of our lives. We need food to survive, of course, but there is meaning to the way we eat, as a social ritual. Many families enjoy sitting down to a meal together every day. We celebrate birthdays, sporting events, and holidays with food. Certain foods have special meaning for us, like pumpkin pie at Thanksgiving or popcorn at the movies.

As the parent of a child with diabetes, you probably have many questions and concerns about what your child can eat. How can you meet your child's dietary needs without disrupting meals for the rest of the family? How can you be sure that she always eats the right foods? Can she eat Halloween candy or birthday cake?

Your family *can* continue to enjoy meals—every day *and* on special occasions. You'll learn new ways to cook old favorites. Healthy eating is important for your child with diabetes and for your whole family. You will find that the extra time you spend planning meals will pay off for everyone.

You will learn to pay close attention to what your child eats and when she eats. Food raises your child's blood glucose. Not enough food can cause blood glucose to drop. Planning meals helps to balance food, insulin, and exercise.

WHY IS MEAL PLANNING IMPORTANT?

Meal planning for children with diabetes is important for two reasons:

■ Your child will get the right amount of calories and nutrients to grow and develop normally.

■ Blood glucose levels will be more easily controlled.

A child's need for nutrients from food depends on age, sex, weight, and activity level. As your child grows, her food needs change. Having a meal plan helps you adjust to these changes in a structured way. It's a good idea to go over your child's meal plan once a year with your dietitian to make sure the plan is still right for your child.

HOW DOES A MEAL PLAN WORK?

Every child's meal plan is different. It depends on what kinds of food your child likes or dislikes, as well as on her age, weight, and so on. Generally, any meal plan for a child with diabetes:

■ provides guidance in planning a healthy diet.

■ includes timing of meals and snacks.

■ guides how much fat, cholesterol, and sugar that your child eats.

■ helps to control your child's diabetes by providing consistent quantities of food so that insulin dosing can also be planned to keep blood glucose levels within a target range. This balance means matching insulin doses to the amount of food to be eaten and insulin action times to eating times.

Having a dietitian as a member of your health care team is very helpful when it comes to meal planning. The dietitian can answer questions or concerns that you or your child may have.

LET APPETITE BE YOUR GUIDE

A child's appetite varies widely and usually indicates the need for food. During growth spurts or times of lots of physical activity, your child may eat heartily. Other times, you may wonder how she keeps going on so little food. Yet, this is the way children normally eat, and having diabetes doesn't change that. You will learn how to make changes in insulin dose based on your child's appetite. It is also important to make meal times pleasant, which means avoiding a battle of wills over food.

When your child was diagnosed with diabetes, she may have lost weight or perhaps not gained weight for a while. Once treatment begins, she may have a tremendous appetite and eat well. After the weight is gained she may not want so much food. Your dietitian will give you a meal plan at diagnosis, but you may need to increase or decrease the number of calories to keep up with her appetite. Therefore, you'll need to keep in touch with your dietitian when making meal plan changes and deciding how much insulin to give to balance the food.

If she's hungry, you can give your child extra food, but do it *at mealtimes*. You can feed her five or six smaller meals throughout the day instead of three large ones, but try to avoid giving extra between-meal snacks. Give your child seconds on foods from all the food groups, not just extra potatoes or bread. On the other hand, if she does not eat well at a meal, try giving a drink such as milk or juice to help keep her blood glucose levels up until the next meal.

A BALANCED DIET

Most people have heard of the four food groups. These days most food experts suggest dividing foods into five groups instead of four:

- grains and breads
- milk and dairy products
- fruits and vegetables
- meat and meat substitutes
- fats and sweets

The three major nutrients our bodies get from food are carbohydrates, protein, and fat. These nutrients do different things in the body.

- Carbohydrates are the body's main source of energy. They are found in fruits, vegetables, bread, cereal, milk, rice, potatoes, and pasta. These foods are turned into glucose during digestion fairly easily, which increases the blood glucose level fairly quickly.
- Protein is used to build and repair body tissue. It is found in meat, poultry, fish, eggs, cheese, peanut butter, and milk. Proteins digest into glucose about half as fast as carbohydrate, causing a slower rise in the blood glucose level that lasts longer.
- Fat provides reserves of energy. It is found in marbled meat, the skin of poultry, whole milk, butter, cheese, and oils such as corn oil and olive oil. It is difficult for the body to turn fat into glucose. Fat has little effect on the blood glucose level other than slowing down the digestion of other nutrients.

If your child eats a wide variety of foods from each of the food groups, vitamin and mineral supplements are usually not necessary.

The meal plan for most children and teens with diabetes is different than for adults with diabetes because children usually don't need to lose weight. Kids need enough calories to grow and develop.

Also, most children and teens do not have heart disease or high blood pressure. Yet, it is well known that people with diabetes are more prone to these difficulties, so although it is not essential to restrict fat and sodium in children and teens, it makes sense to be prudent about it. Eating less fat and salt can help to reduce the risk of developing these problems. Healthy eating guidelines developed by the U.S. government advise Americans to cut the fat in their diets to no more than 30% of all calories they eat. The American Diabetes Association, along with The American Dietetic Association, has written its own dietary guidelines that agree with those of the U.S. government. The Diabetes Food Guide Pyramid on the next page can help you to see that your whole family eats a healthy diet. Your dietitian or other health care provider can help you to plan meals that are both healthy and enjoyable.

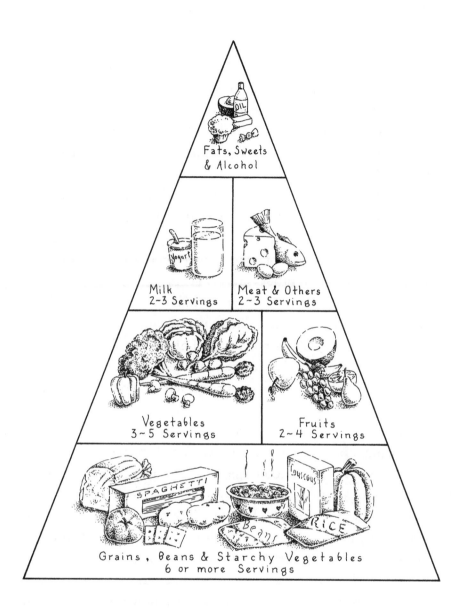

Fats, Sweets & Alcohol

Milk
2–3 Servings

Meat & Others
2–3 Servings

Vegetables
3–5 Servings

Fruits
2–4 Servings

Grains, Beans & Starchy Vegetables
6 or more Servings

Carbohydrates and Sugars

As you know, glucose is the body's main energy source. Before it can be used as energy, glucose must get inside the body's cells. Insulin is the key that opens the cell doors, letting the glucose in. People with type 1 diabetes don't make insulin, so glucose stays in their blood instead of entering the cells. Glucose comes from food that is eaten, mostly from carbohydrates.

Carbohydrates are found in fruits, vegetables, bread, cereal, milk, rice, potatoes, and pasta. Foods like bread, potatoes, and pasta are called starches or complex carbohydrates. The body breaks them down into glucose. It takes a little more time to break down complex carbohydrates into glucose than carbohydrates that are closer in form to glucose, such as candy, table sugar, and fruit juice.

Sugar. Sugar (sucrose) is a carbohydrate. For many years, health professionals thought that people with diabetes should avoid foods that contain sugar. We now know, however, that foods that contain sugar, when eaten as part of a meal, have about the same effect on blood glucose levels as other carbohydrates. For example, a dessert brownie that has 15 grams of sugar will affect your child's blood glucose level about the same as a dinner potato with margarine, which has about 15 grams of carbohydrate. This means that foods containing sugar can be part of your child's meal plan as long as:

- they are eaten in small amounts (preferably with a complete meal)
- your child's blood glucose levels are checked regularly
- you monitor the total amount of carbohydrate in your child's diet

It's a good idea to encourage your child to eat only a small amount of sugary foods. Most of these foods have little nutritional value and they are often high in fat. Talk to your dietitian about the best way to fit some sugary foods into your child's meal plan.

Fruits and fruit juice. Fruits and fruit juice contain natural sugar (fructose), but they also contain fiber and other important nutrients. Your dietitian will recommend how much fruit your child with diabetes should eat at each meal or snack.

Sugary foods usually make blood glucose rise quickly. Complex carbohydrates and protein usually make it rise more slowly and can prevent it from dropping again. That's why it's a good idea to give your child something sweet, followed by a sandwich or crackers with cheese or peanut butter when her blood glucose is low. (See page 81.)

At certain times you may want to give your child fruit juice or a sugary food in order to raise her blood glucose. The following are examples of times when you may want to do this:

■ to balance a low blood glucose reading
■ during or after exercise
■ during a long gap between meals
■ on sick days if blood glucose is low

Fat and Cholesterol

Unless your child is younger than 2, her meal plan limits the amount of fat and cholesterol that she eats. The U.S. government's healthy eating guidelines advise all Americans over age 2 to eat less fat (especially saturated fat) and cholesterol to reduce the chances of getting heart disease.

Saturated fat and cholesterol are found mostly in animal products, including butter, lard, whole milk, and fatty meats. Using low-fat milk and cheese and eating lean meat will help you and your child to eat less saturated fat.

HOW DO I DO MEAL PLANNING?

Meal plans generally include three meals and two or three snacks a day. It is a good idea for your child to eat at about the same time most days. Meals and snacks are planned to balance the way insulin works in your child's body.

But your child's schedule won't be the same every day. Gym class at school may be changed to a different time. Going out on a family picnic may mean eating lunch later than usual. It's okay to adjust your child's meal plan when your child's or the family's schedule changes. For example, when you know that a meal is going to be eaten later than usual, make sure your child eats a snack to keep her blood glucose from getting too low.

There are many ways to do meal planning for children with diabetes. What's right for your child depends on the kind of foods she likes to eat, as well as on her age, appetite, weight, and activity level. Your health care provider can help you to find what works best for your child.

What Are Exchanges?

Exchanges are one way of making meal planning easier for people with diabetes. Your doctor or dietitian can give you a booklet

---

PLANNING MEALS USING EXCHANGES

The following are examples of meals you might plan for your child using the Exchange Lists (2,200-calorie plan)

Breakfast: 1 milk, 1 fruit, 2 starches, and 2 meats
1 cup (8 oz) fat-free (skim) milk (1 milk)
half-cup (4 oz) orange juice (1 fruit)
2 slices of bread (2 starches)
2 slices of lean ham (2 meats)

Lunch: 3 starches, 2 meats, 1 fruit, 1 milk, and 3 fats
grilled cheese sandwich (2 starches, 2 meats, 1 fat)
small apple (1 fruit)
1 cup (8 oz) fat-free (skim) milk (1 milk)
1 oz pretzels (1 starch)

Afternoon snack: 1 starch, 1 milk
3 cups air-popped popcorn (1 starch)
1 cup (8 oz) fat-free yogurt (1 milk)

Dinner: 3 starches, 3 meats, 1 fruit, 1 milk, 2 fats, and 2 vegetables
salad with 1 Tbsp dressing (1 vegetable, 1 fat)
medium potato (1 starch)
3 oz baked chicken (3 meats)
2-inch roll (1 starch)
green beans (1 vegetable)
baked apple (1 fruit)
1 cup (8 oz) fat-free (skim) milk (1 milk)

Bedtime snack: 1 starch, 1 meat, and 1 milk
1/2 turkey sandwich (1 starch, 1 meat)
1 cup (8 oz) fat-free (skim) milk (1 milk)

---

called *Exchange Lists for Meal Planning* that explains how to plan meals using exchanges. This booklet divides foods into lists, including:

∎ starches

∎ meats

∎ vegetables

∎ fruits

∎ milk

∎ fat

A food on any one of these lists can be exchanged, or traded, for any other food on the same list. Your child's individual meal plan tells you how many portions, or exchanges, can be chosen from each list at a meal. Using exchanges helps to make sure that your child eats the right amounts of nutrients every day.

Carbohydrate Counting

Another approach to meal planning is to count the number of carbohydrates in the food consumed. A dietitian will give you guidance about how much carbohydrate to include for meals and snacks. By counting how many carbohydrates are consumed, you can determine how much insulin to give.

> Jodi should eat a total of 60 grams of carbohydrate for breakfast. She can have the total all in waffles, or she can have cereal, milk, and fruit, as long as the total comes to around 60. She knows that if she eats 60 grams of carbohydrate she needs about 4 units of insulin at breakfast.

You will need to know how sensitive your child's body is to carbohydrate. This means figuring out how much carbohydrate 1 unit of insulin can take care of. A unit of insulin may cover 20 grams of carbohydrate in one person but less than 10 grams of carbohydrate in another.

To find this out, your child will need to monitor her blood glucose levels before and after meals, count carbohydrate totals in each meal, and relate them to units of insulin taken before each meal. Then you can figure out about how many units of insulin will cover a certain amount of carbohydrate. This diabetes management tool is for kids and their parents who like math!

This system can work well for people doing intensive diabetes management with either multiple daily injections or an insulin pump. Both of these types of diabetes management are better for older children, over 7 or 8 years old. The dietitian on your health care team can show you how to get started counting carbohydrates.

Alternative Sweeteners

Alternative sweeteners are products that can be used instead of sugar to sweeten food. People with diabetes can safely use alternative sweeteners. Most (but not all) alternative sweeteners have few calories. Some alternative sweeteners now available include:

- **Saccharin** is about 400 times as sweet as sugar. People with diabetes can safely use saccharin. A possible disadvantage of saccharin is that it can leave a slightly bitter aftertaste.
- **Aspartame** is about 200 times as sweet as sugar. Most people, including people with diabetes, can safely use aspartame. However, aspartame is not safe for people who have a rare condition called phenylketonuria (PKU). Aspartame can't be used for cooking because it breaks down when heated.
- **Acesulfame-K** contains natural flavors extracted from fruits. It can be used safely by people with diabetes or PKU.
- **Sucralose** is a good choice for cooking or baking.
- **Fructose** (fruit sugar) is naturally found in fruit, so it is not calorie-free like other artificial sweeteners. It is a carbohydrate that is broken down by the body more slowly than other sugars. Fructose should be counted as carbohydrate in a meal plan for diabetes. In an exchange diet, it is counted as a fruit exchange.

BECOMING A FOOD DETECTIVE

In spite of efforts to be consistent in the amounts of carbohydrates eaten, there are differences in how quickly these foods are used by the body. Different foods affect people in various ways. You may begin to notice that some foods affect your child's blood glucose level more than others. For example, eating spaghetti may make her blood glucose run higher than eating mashed potatoes and meat loaf. Waffles for breakfast may cause a rise in blood glucose before lunch, but cereal may not. Pizza prepared at different places may have different effects on blood glucose.

This doesn't mean that your child can't eat those foods. As you become aware of the effects that different foods have, you can use this knowledge to balance these foods with insulin or exercise. For example, if you know that crackers make your child's blood glucose run higher than pretzels, you may want to pack crackers for her snack on a day when she is going skating. If waffles make her blood glucose run high, you know that your child will need extra insulin on waffle days.

Keeping a daily log of what your child eats can help you identify how different foods affect your child's blood glucose. You can use this food diary to adjust your child's insulin dosage depending on what she is eating.

This sort of detective work takes time and effort. The reward is that you and your child have more control over her diabetes. Your dietitian and diabetes educator can help you become skilled at this kind of analysis.

Joanna's glucose always runs high when she eats pizza. So, on days when Joanna's mother knows she is going to be eating pizza, she gives her a bit more insulin than usual to maintain balance.

HOW CAN I HELP MY CHILD
TO ACCEPT MEAL PLANNING?

Even though your child's meal plan can be flexible enough to work in a favorite food or dessert, there may be times when you don't want your child to eat what everyone else is eating so she can have better blood glucose control. These decisions can be difficult, because as a parent you want your child to feel part of the group and not have feelings about being different. However, just like children who have food allergies, there are times when it is not in your child's best interest to eat a particular food.

One of the best approaches is to stay positive and flexible about food choices, while realizing that there will be times when you must say "No!" to your child. There may be other times where you allow the food choice with the understanding that her blood glucose just might have to run high for a period of time.

The best approach to meal planning, though, is to figure out a way that your child can have what she wants and still keep her blood glucose levels in her range. Your child's health and safety is a primary concern, but diabetes is a lifelong condition, and feeling too deprived or different as a child can cause long-term resistance to diabetes management.

Each situation that comes up may be different, and you will need to have the skills and understanding to make decisions along the way. How you decide to do this depends on the situation, the timing of the food, whether you are able to make an adjustment in insulin easily, your child's frame of mind about the food or situation, and her blood glucose level.

Try to include your child in the decision. For example, if your child's blood glucose level is running high and she really doesn't care that much for the chocolate cake being served, you may decide together to go with the usual meal plan that day and skip the cake. Or, if she feels strongly about eating the cake, you may work out a compromise.

As your child grows and learns about diabetes, it will be important that she understands about food groups and carbohydrates and how they affect her blood glucose levels. Learning this will take time and patience, but it will allow her to make her own decisions about when to choose pretzels over a cupcake, or how to adjust if she eats the cupcake.

It is helpful if everyone in the family eats the same meal instead of serving a separate meal for the child with diabetes. That way, there's no reason for the child with diabetes to feel different. Besides, a meal that is healthy for a person with diabetes is healthy for everyone.

Sometimes your child can have food that looks a lot like the food others are eating. For example, when her friends are having fried hamburgers, potato chips, and cola, your child can have a broiled hamburger, pretzels, and a diet soda. Your child's food is similar to her friends' food, but it is lower in fat and sugar.

With a bit of planning, your child can have lunch at school with her friends. Many schools give out copies of lunch menus to help parents who need to plan their children's meals ahead of time. By using these menus, you can help your child choose foods that fit in with her meal plan.

Involving your child in planning meals and snacks is always smart. She may find it easier to follow a meal plan that she has helped to influence.

Some children may go through a phase of hiding candy in their school locker or having a cookie and ice cream binge after school. Your child may be rebelling at feeling different, or testing to see what will happen if she eats whatever she wants.

Try to maintain open communication with her if she's having difficulty. If after learning about these behaviors you can maintain your composure rather than becoming upset or punitive, it will help your child trust that she can share this information with you.

Ask her to let you know if or when she snacks on sweets because this information will help you to adjust her insulin. Help her to understand the consequences of ignoring her meal plan, both short and long term (she will feel too ill to play after school; she may have complications later—see page 94).

Having a meal plan that is flexible and includes some sweets may prevent your child from bingeing or sneaking food. Then praise her with positive reinforcement when she follows her meal plan.

Seven-year-old Amy's blood test results were often high when she came home from school. Her parents suspected eating extra treats on the school bus caused the problem. Her mother put Amy on her lap, hugged her, and asked her if she was eating candy with her friends. Amy admitted that she was. She said she wanted to join in with what her friends were doing. Amy and her mother talked about how hard it was not for her to eat candy when her friends were eating it. Her mother explained that eating too many candies made Amy's glucose high and that high glucose made Amy feel thirsty and tired. In the end they decided that Amy should take small boxes of raisins with her to share with her friends on the school bus. She could eat the raisins and feel like one of the gang. After that, Amy's after-school blood test results improved.

COPING WITH SCHEDULE CHANGES

A schedule change will sometimes prevent your child from following her usual meal plan. If sticking to the meal plan means singling her out and upsetting her, it may be better to adjust the meal plan for the schedule change. However, your child's diabetes control may not be the best on these occasions.

A special event at school may mean that the time of your child's lunch hour or gym class is changed for a few days. If you know about this change ahead of time, you can add a snack to the meal plan or adjust the insulin dose to maintain balance. It can help to talk with your child's teachers and ask them to inform you whenever there is a change to the school schedule that affects your child's meal times or exercise routine, so you can plan ahead. (See *Communicating with Your Child's School and Teachers,* page 111.)

If lunch is delayed for more than an hour for some reason, giving your child any food that contains about 15 grams of carbohydrate (such as 6 low-fat crackers, 2 pretzels, or 3 graham crackers) will prevent low blood glucose. Additional snacks are helpful anytime your child gets extra exercise or has to wait longer than usual between meals.

HOLIDAYS AND PARTIES

Holidays are extra-special times for children, and eating is often a central part of holiday celebrations. Usually the food is plentiful and there are lots of special sweet dishes. Having diabetes need not prevent your child from enjoying these special occasions. With careful planning, she can eat most of the same foods that everyone else is eating.

The classic difficulty here is that holidays can occur over several days or even weeks. Try to limit the food extravagances to the actual day of the holiday instead of the whole holiday season. Or arrange other types of treats, like small toys or extra privileges, for each day of the season.

Plan ahead so that extra foods, such as Grandma's special pie, baked goods, and candy, can be covered with extra insulin. Otherwise, help your child to stick to her meal plan. Try some of the following hints to help your child focus on the festivities instead of the food.

■ **Easter:** Fill an Easter basket with treats other than food, such as coloring books or stickers, clothing or jewelry. Or fill plastic eggs with promises of treats, like a chance to stay up late or a trip to a museum or to the movies.

■ **Halloween:** Have your child trade that trick-or-treat bag full of sweets for a present she has been wanting. Or auction it off to the rest of the family for spending money. Instead of trick-

or-treating, collect money for a good cause. Or take a trip to visit a haunted house or see a scary movie. Suggest gum, pretzels, nuts, granola bars, or raisins as treats to friends and neighbors. Allow your child to choose a handful of favorite Halloween candy to save for special treats.

■ **Thanksgiving, Christmas, or Hanukkah:** The holiday dinner is not usually a problem, although extra insulin may be needed. However, in some families, the meal falls mid-afternoon. There are several ways to approach an unusual schedule, so it is important to talk to your diabetes educator to decide the best way to cover the meal with insulin. Harder to deal with are the sweets and goodies that may be available for days. Talk to your child about having one treat she really likes with her meal, and balance her insulin and exercise accordingly. Keep tempting treats out of reach during the day.

The excitement of holidays can affect children's blood glucose levels. For example, the thrill of opening presents on Christmas morning can distract a child from eating and cause low blood glucose. You can adjust for this by reducing insulin or reminding your child to eat.

When your child does eat sweets, try to problem-solve how much insulin it takes to cover the extra food. You can do this by finding out how many grams of carbohydrate are in the food, having your child test her blood glucose, giving her a certain amount

---

Jodi wants to eat a soft ice cream cone on the Fourth of July. Help her find out how much carbohydrate is in the ice cream and cone. Have her test her blood glucose. Then, give her insulin based on the number of grams of carbohydrate and her blood glucose level. Jodi then eats the ice cream, and tests her blood 2 hours later. If her blood glucose is high after 2 hours, she should take more insulin the next time she wants the cone.

Seven-year-old Ashleigh is going to a birthday party from 6 to 8 p.m. The party theme is a tea party, with very little activity planned. Ashleigh wants to enjoy the birthday cake that will be served at the party. Cake always makes her glucose levels high. Ashleigh gets regular insulin every day before dinner at 5 p.m. Her mother gives her an extra unit of regular insulin with her predinner injection on the day of the party. Ashleigh can now enjoy the birthday cake and still prevent her glucose levels from going too high.

of insulin, having her eat the food, then testing again 2 hours later. Your doctor, nurse, or dietitian can help with this. Usually, 15 grams of carbohydrate is the equivalent of about 1 unit of insulin for teens and adults.

Many party foods are sweet and high in fat. If your child is going to a party, you may want to get in touch with the hosts beforehand to find out what kind of food is being served.

If a lot of high-fat, high-sugar foods are on the menu, you may want to offer to bring some healthier choices. For example, popcorn or cereal snacks can substitute for candy at a child's birthday party. Most parents will welcome the offer.

It's okay for your child to eat birthday cake or other party foods. It's worth some planning ahead to help keep your child from feeling left out. Before your child goes to a party, it's smart to make plans with her about how she wants to eat and why. Then you can try some options:

■ Talk to her about scraping off some of the cake icing to reduce the amount of carbohydrate she eats.

■ Adjust insulin or alter the amount of food at other meals or the timing of meals to account for the party foods. Sometimes the extra food is substituted for a snack or part of a meal. At other times, it's eaten in addition to the child's usual food.

■ Plan a calorie-burning family outing after the party.

Your diabetes educator can help you to plan for special events. The box below provides some ideas for children's parties that your child with diabetes can enjoy.

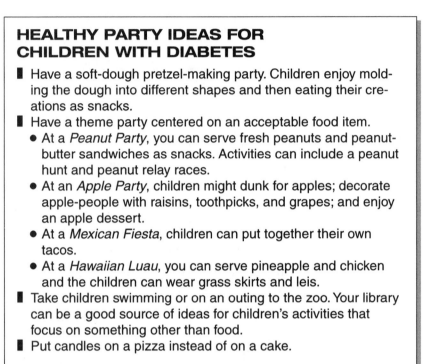

HEALTHY PARTY IDEAS FOR CHILDREN WITH DIABETES

- Have a soft-dough pretzel-making party. Children enjoy molding the dough into different shapes and then eating their creations as snacks.
- Have a theme party centered on an acceptable food item.
  - At a *Peanut Party*, you can serve fresh peanuts and peanut-butter sandwiches as snacks. Activities can include a peanut hunt and peanut relay races.
  - At an *Apple Party*, children might dunk for apples; decorate apple-people with raisins, toothpicks, and grapes; and enjoy an apple dessert.
  - At a *Mexican Fiesta*, children can put together their own tacos.
  - At a *Hawaiian Luau*, you can serve pineapple and chicken and the children can wear grass skirts and leis.
- Take children swimming or on an outing to the zoo. Your library can be a good source of ideas for children's activities that focus on something other than food.
- Put candles on a pizza instead of on a cake.

EATING OUT

Like other special occasions involving food, eating out can be safe and enjoyable for people with diabetes. Many restaurants and fast food chains can provide information on the calorie and fat content of menu items. Some offer exchange lists to make meal planning easier. Ask questions about things on the menu. Most restaurant staff will be happy to answer your questions.

Eating away from home means food won't always show up when you expect it. If your meal is taking longer to appear on the table than you planned and you're worried about your child's blood glucose dropping low, ask for some rolls (go easy on the butter) or crackers or a soft drink. If you're at an event where you're not sure when food will be served, such as a wedding reception, think about waiting to inject insulin until you know that food is within reach.

HELPFUL HINTS FOR EATING OUT

- Ask if food is breaded or fried before ordering it.
- Request that meats be broiled rather than fried.
- Ask if sauces are sweetened.
- Request that dishes be served without butter, fats, or oils.
- Ask that salad dressings, margarine, sour cream, and sauces be served on the side.
- Ask for lite or sugar-free syrup, jelly, or dressing.

If you think your child's soft drink isn't sugar-free:

Sometimes you may not be sure that the diet soda you ordered is really sugar-free. To find out, try dipping a urine test strip into the drink. If the strip turns dark, there is probably sugar in the drink. Most sugar-free soft drinks will not cause the strip to turn dark. But drinks made from sugar-free powdered mixes (such as sugar-free Kool-Aid and iced tea mixes) will change the strips because they contain small amounts of substances similar to sugar. You may want to play it safe by ordering a canned drink that you know is sugar-free. Sometimes, drinks from a fountain can be mixed up.

Playing Games and Sports Safely

When children first develop diabetes they may wonder, "Can I still play with my friends or go out for sports?" The answer is definitely yes. Reassure your child that professional athletes with diabetes have played in all the national leagues.

All children should be encouraged to be physically active, and children with diabetes are no exception. Regular exercise has many benefits:

- It strengthens the heart and lungs.
- It builds muscle and improves flexibility in the joints.
- It builds confidence and reduces stress.
- It provides interaction with other children.

For people with diabetes physical activity has an added benefit: it helps to lower blood glucose levels. When the body's muscles are working, more glucose moves into muscle tissue instead of staying in the blood. Children who exercise regularly usually need less insulin than other kids do. (But be sure to consult with your doctor before initiating any change in your child's insulin dose.) Taking part in gym class and team sports also helps your child to develop social skills, make friends, and feel like one of the gang.

Although exercise has not been shown to make blood glucose control easier, it is still an important and necessary part of treating diabetes. Because it is difficult to estimate how much food is required to cover a certain amount of exercise, children who exercise strenuously often find that blood glucose numbers vary considerably. It is important, however, to learn how to manage the effect of exercise by doing frequent monitoring of blood glucose.

Getting *regular* exercise is important for people with diabetes because of the need to balance the effect of exercise with food and insulin. Activities that meet regularly, like swimming or soccer, make it easier to plan meals and insulin doses.

This chapter provides general guidance on making physical activity and exercise as safe as possible for children with diabetes. If you have specific questions about what's right for your child, check with your doctor or diabetes educator.

BEING PREPARED FOR UNPLANNED GAMES AND ACTIVITIES

Your health care provider can help you to make regular, planned exercise an enjoyable and safe part of your child's life. But children's lives also involve a lot of unplanned activity. For example, your child may take part in a spontaneous basketball game or some other strenuous activity with friends.

Because exercise lowers blood glucose levels, unplanned physical activity may cause your child's blood glucose to drop. The simplest way to prevent this is to have him always carry snack foods like crackers with peanut butter or cheese, which contain carbohydrate and protein to boost blood glucose levels. It's a good idea for your child to eat a snack before taking part in any unplanned physical activity.

Depending on how strenuous the activity is, additional snacks may be needed during the play or afterward. These snacks are eaten in addition to the child's usual meals. They replace the glucose that the muscle cells use during exercise.

How much food your child needs to eat depends on what his blood glucose level is and how strenuous the activity is. By checking blood glucose levels before the activity, you and your child can decide how much extra food is needed.

GUIDELINES FOR SNACKS AND EXERCISE

The following are general guidelines for snacks before exercise. A dietitian may suggest other guidelines for your child. Consult your health care provider for specific advice.

Light activities (such as walking, bowling, or ping-pong)
Carbohydrate need: 20–30 grams per hour of exercise
Blood glucose 70–180 mg/dl: 3–5 pretzels or 2–3 cups of pop-corn would provide 10–15 grams of carbohydrate
Blood glucose over 180 mg/dl: A snack may not be required before light exercise, or it can be eaten after the exercise.

Vigorous activities (such as jogging or competitive swimming)
Carbohydrate need: 30–60 grams per hour of exercise
Blood glucose 70–180 mg/dl: 1–2 sandwiches or 1 sandwich and 1 fruit eaten before exercise provides enough complex carbo-hydrate and protein for 1 hour of strenuous exercise.
Blood glucose above 180 mg/dl: 1 sandwich or 1 fruit

WHAT ELSE CAN I DO TO BE SURE MY CHILD CAN ALWAYS PLAY SAFELY?

As well as carrying snack foods like crackers or pretzels, it's a good idea for youngsters to carry a backup source of glucose to guard against lows. Always keep a package of sugar cubes, hard candy, or glucose tablets in your child's backpack, purse, or pocket.

One athletic youngster keeps a pack of glucose tablets in his football helmet so it's available during a game if he needs it. Some parents buy their children gym shorts and sweat suits with pockets so they can carry sugary snacks.

Talk with your child's gym teachers and sports coaches about the symptoms of low blood glucose and what to do if it occurs (see page 78). It's important that your child exercise with a buddy whenever possible in case he has an episode of low blood glucose and needs help. Make sure the buddy knows what to do or how to get help.

Lengthy exercise (like a day-long ski trip) or a major change in routine (like the start of football training) requires special planning. Talk to your health care provider about how to prepare for these kinds of activities.

Strenuous exercise like jogging or swimming laps can affect glucose levels up to 24 hours later. Even if your child snacks before strenuous exercise, he may still have low blood glucose afterward. It's generally suggested that blood glucose be checked during the night on a day when the child has had more exercise than usual.

BALANCING EXERCISE AND INSULIN

What if you take all these precautions and your child still has lows during gym class or while playing games? If that happens, your child's insulin dosage may need to be decreased.

Insulin may also need to be decreased if your child is taking part in a vigorous sport like swimming, soccer, or football, and doesn't want to load up on food beforehand. Big changes in your child's insulin dosage should only be made after discussion with your doctor. You can, however, learn how to fine-tune your child's dosage to control glucose levels. (See *Adjusting Insulin at Home*, page 38.)

Children should not exercise if ketones are present in their urine. Ketones can be a sign that there is too little insulin available. Exercise causes fat to be broken down and can increase the amount of ketones in the body. (See *Urine Testing*, page 47.)

PRECAUTIONS FOR
SAFE PHYSICAL ACTIVITY

Before exercise

∎ check blood glucose level
∎ eat an extra carbohydrate-rich snack

At all times

∎ carry sugar cubes or glucose tablets to treat lows
∎ don't exercise if ketones are present in the urine
∎ during strenuous exercise, stop every 30 minutes to eat or drink a carbohydrate-rich snack
∎ exercise with a buddy if possible

The Highs and Lows of Diabetes

As a general rule, you can consider your child's diabetes to be reasonably well-controlled if her blood glucose level is within the target range most of the time and she does not get severe symptoms of low blood glucose.

Sometimes, however, insulin, food, and exercise are not balanced and your child may show signs of high or low blood glucose. Eating different amounts or different types of food or being more or less active than usual will affect your child's blood glucose levels. Differences in the way the body absorbs insulin or the presence of other hormones that respond to insulin may also cause blood glucose levels to be too high or too low.

Most of the time you'll be aware in advance of situations that might cause high or low blood glucose. Sometimes, however, it can happen for no apparent reason. Knowing how to identify high and low blood glucose levels, and what to do when they happen, can help you to act quickly to protect your child's health.

HYPOGLYCEMIA (LOW BLOOD GLUCOSE)

Hypoglycemia is the most common problem in children with diabetes. Most of the time it is mild and can be easily treated by giving the child something sweet.

Food raises blood glucose levels and insulin and exercise lower them. Low blood glucose can occur when the balance of insulin, food, and exercise is upset. The body can't control insulin that's given as an injection in the same way it controls insulin that the body makes itself. Once an injection is given, the insulin can't be stopped or slowed down. So if too much insulin is available, blood glucose levels will drop too low.

People with diabetes have to control their own blood glucose levels because the ability to regulate insulin is gone. Eating meals and getting insulin injections at regular times and snacking before exercise help to prevent glucose levels from dropping too low.

Hypoglycemia must be treated promptly to prevent blood glucose levels from getting so low that the brain is deprived of glucose. Too little glucose in the brain can cause severe symptoms, such as:

▌ sleepiness and unresponsiveness

▌ seizures

▌ unconsciousness

How Can I Tell If My Child's Blood Glucose Is Low?

The symptoms of low blood glucose may be different each time it happens. Sometimes your child may have no obvious symptoms. For these reasons, it is a good idea to teach a child with diabetes to tell you whenever she feels strange in any way.

In children under 3, misbehavior or crankiness may be a sign that the child's blood glucose is low. Very young children can't tell you when they're not feeling well, so you need to be on the lookout for warning signs. Frequent blood glucose tests can help to relieve anxiety when you aren't certain what is going on.

Most parents learn to recognize the symptoms of low blood glucose in their children. It is a good idea to talk with your child's

A quick-witted teacher reported this experience with a usually pleasant and calm student. While waiting in the cafeteria line at lunch, the youngster became irritable and punched a classmate for no reason. The teacher guessed that the cause of the behavior might be low blood glucose and gave the student a glass of orange juice and some crackers. In about 15 minutes, after the juice and crackers began to raise her blood glucose level, the student became her usual pleasant self again.

teachers (and other adults with whom your child has contact) about the symptoms of low blood glucose.

Scientists think that low blood glucose may continue to affect a child's learning ability for awhile (perhaps an hour or more) after it has been treated. A period when your child's glucose level is low may not be the best time for her to take an important exam or give a presentation. This is another reason why it's a good idea to talk to your child's teachers about low blood glucose.

Sometimes your child may feel nervous, anxious, or tired and think it's because of low blood glucose. She may have some of the symptoms of low blood glucose if her glucose level drops quickly from high to normal. The best thing to do if you or your child suspect that blood glucose is low is to do a blood test.

If the child has symptoms of low blood glucose but the blood test shows that glucose isn't low, repeat the test. She may be experiencing a fast drop in blood glucose without being in any danger of hypoglycemia. Giving her a few crackers to eat should help the low feelings subside and are not harmful. In a few minutes she can return to her normal activities.

If In Doubt, Treat. If you think your child may have low blood glucose but you can't do a blood test right away, give your child something sweet to eat. The treatment will not do any harm even if the child's glucose level is not low.

Three-year-old Jenny was at the shopping mall with her grand-mother. Her grandmother knew that it was getting close to Jenny's lunchtime, but she only had one more errand. Jenny became very irritable and had a temper tantrum at the check-out line. Her grandmother didn't know if Jenny had a tantrum because she refused to buy a toy that Jenny wanted or she was having a problem with low blood glucose. Her grandmother real-ized that she had forgotten Jenny's testing meter in the car. Her grandmother decided to give Jenny a juice box to sip just in case her glucose was low.

Preventing Low Blood Glucose

It's important to prevent low blood glucose because frequent or unrecognized episodes can lead to more severe, potentially dan-gerous events.

Low blood glucose can usually be prevented by:

■ testing glucose levels regularly

■ following the recommended meal plan

■ making sure the insulin dose is correct

■ eating extra snacks before exercise that is unplanned or more strenuous than usual

You may need to remind your child that testing blood glucose helps to make sure that the insulin dose and meal plan are right. Your child's insulin dose or meal plan may need to be changed if your child has frequent episodes.

If you and your child are trying to keep her glucose levels near normal, you can expect that she will have mild episodes of low blood glucose occasionally. While not desirable, they are proba-bly not dangerous and are easily treated.

Treating Low Blood Glucose:
Mild to Moderate Symptoms

Low blood glucose needs to be treated quickly. The way to treat it is to give your child a sweet food like glucose tablets, fruit juice, soda, or raisins, followed by four crackers. A candy bar is not the best choice because its high fat content may not raise blood glucose quickly. But if a candy bar is the only food available, it is an alternative treatment for low blood glucose.

It may take 10 to 20 minutes for her blood glucose level to rise, depending on how much food is already in your child's stomach. If she isn't feeling better in 20 minutes, check her blood glucose level again. If it's still low, repeat the treatment.

A low blood glucose episode may occur just before a snack or a meal. If this happens, give your child something sweet and see that she eats the snack or meal as soon as possible.

If snack or mealtime isn't close, give your child a snack food containing complex carbohydrate and protein after the sweet food. Crackers with cheese or peanut butter, cereal and milk, or half a sandwich are good choices. This food is eaten in addition to the day's usual meals.

> David was going on a long hike with a group of children. His mother told the counselor in charge to give David something sweet if he showed symptoms of low blood glucose. When David felt shaky at the beginning of the hike, the counselor gave him sugar cubes. Twenty minutes later David felt shaky again. The counselor gave him more sugar cubes. This happened every 20 minutes during the trip. To prevent this chain of events, the counselor could have given David a complex carbohydrate and protein (such as a cheese or peanut butter sandwich) at the beginning of the hike.

Treating Low Blood Glucose: Severe Symptoms

A child who is very drowsy, unconscious, or unable to eat, drink, or swallow may be experiencing severe low blood glucose.

Do *not* put anything in your child's mouth if she is unconscious, as she could choke or clamp down on your fingers. If she can't or won't swallow, you will need to give her an injection of *glucagon* to raise blood glucose levels. Glucagon is a hormone normally made by the pancreas. Your doctor should give you a prescription so that you can always have glucagon on hand. Make sure you know how to use it. The injection usually takes effect within 15 to 20 minutes. If the child does not respond within that time, contact your doctor or take the child to an emergency room right away. A common side effect after taking glucagon is vomiting. Tell your doctor about the shot—changes may need to be made in insulin doses.

> Paul's father heard him crying in his sleep. His dad went to check on Paul and found him to be pale, sweaty, and difficult to awaken. He tried to get Paul to swallow some juice, but Paul was shaking and was not cooperative. Paul's father gave him an injection of glucagon, and within minutes Paul was awake.

Being Prepared for Low Blood Glucose Emergencies

It's a good idea for everyone who takes insulin to always carry something sweet for emergencies. Packages of glucose tablets, sugar cubes, or candy are useful because they are easy to carry. It's also a good idea to carry a sandwich, cheese or peanut butter crackers, or some other food containing complex carbohydrate and protein.

Keep a glucagon kit at home in a place everyone knows about, such as the refrigerator butter keeper. Check the expiration date on the kit periodically. Also keep a travel kit for use in case of severe low blood glucose. Be sure that school personnel, baby-sitters, and others who take care of your child know how to use glucagon, too.

Adults caring for a child with diabetes often are afraid to treat symptoms of low blood glucose because they think that eating

TREATING LOW BLOOD GLUCOSE

Mild to moderate symptoms (child is alert and can swallow)

Treat right away with a sweet food:

1/2–3/4 cup orange or apple juice
1–2 glucose tablets or doses of glucose gel
2–4 LifeSavers (or similar product)
5 small gumdrops
1–2 Tbsp honey
6 oz nondiet soda
2 Tbsp cake icing (such as decorator icing gel in a tube)

Follow a few minutes later with:

2–4 soda crackers and 1 oz of cheese, OR
1 Tbsp peanut butter (or other complex carbohydrate and protein)

Don't overtreat! One-half cup (4 oz) of orange juice or a glucose drink, followed by 4 crackers, should be enough to relieve symptoms. Remember that sugar takes time to be absorbed. Give more sugar after about 15 minutes if the symptoms don't go away.

Severe symptoms (child is very sleepy, very shaky, unconscious, or unable to eat, drink, or swallow)

Treat immediately with an injection of glucagon. The standard dose is 1 mg. However, children up to age 6 usually only need 0.5 mg (half the standard dose). The injection should take effect in 15–20 minutes. If the child doesn't respond, call your doctor or take the child to an emergency room.

sweets will harm the child. Be sure that your child's teachers, coaches, and babysitters understand the symptoms of low blood glucose and know that sugar is the proper treatment.

Remember: check blood glucose if you're not sure whether your child is low. But if you can't test, treat with something sweet.

Should My Child Wear a Medical ID Tag?

It's a good idea for everyone who has diabetes, including young children, to wear a medical identification tag at all times. These tags can save lives in an emergency.

The kind of tag you choose will depend on your child's age and preference. It is most important that the tag be in a style your child will wear. For young children, ankle chains are probably the best choice. Neck chains are not suitable for infants and preschoolers, who are likely to play with the chains and may break them or choke on them.

A variety of colorful nylon bracelets are available for children. Teenagers may prefer a necklace-style chain. Sewing ID tags into the child's undershirts is another option.

Makers and styles of medical ID tags change frequently. Ask your diabetes educator or pharmacist for a current list of suppliers or see the *Diabetes Forecast Resource Guide*, published every January by the American Diabetes Association.

Wallet cards also are helpful, as they carry your child's medical information. You can get wallet cards in most pharmacies and from your local chapter of the American Diabetes Association.

HYPERGLYCEMIA (HIGH BLOOD GLUCOSE)

Blood glucose levels can rise when your child gets too little insulin or too much food, or when she is less active than usual. Physical and emotional stress can also cause blood glucose levels to rise. Having a cold or sore throat, an injury, worrying about exams, family crises, poor insulin absorption, or going through the hormonal changes of puberty may all cause hyperglycemia.

Preventing and Treating Hyperglycemia

When blood glucose is high, there is an imbalance between the amount of food, exercise, and insulin present. Sticking to a meal plan is one of the best ways to keep within the target range. However, even then, sometimes blood glucose levels run high.

One of the most helpful strategies to prevent high blood glucose levels is to do frequent monitoring and keep records. Then you often can figure out how to prevent the high the next time. (See *Nitty-Gritty 2—Glucose Testing*, page 43.) This will enable you to adjust your child's insulin dose, food intake, or exercise level to prevent symptoms from occurring.

Unless a child is overweight and trying to shed pounds, it's not a good idea to cut down on food to lower glucose levels. Your child needs food to grow and develop normally. Her meal plan is designed to give her the nutrients she needs. Spacing meals and snacks farther apart may help if your child often gets high blood glucose, but talk this over with your doctor or diabetes educator before trying it. Mild exercise can also help to bring a moderately elevated (under 300 mg/dl) blood glucose down.

KETOACIDOSIS AND DIABETIC COMA

Ketones are acid waste products that are created when the body burns fat to get the energy it needs. They build up in the blood and spill into the urine. Very high levels of ketones in the blood and urine lead to a condition called *ketoacidosis*.

Ketoacidosis is a very serious condition. Diabetic coma can be a result of severe or prolonged ketoacidosis. A person can have ketoacidosis without being in a coma, though. Untreated, ketoacidosis is life-threatening.

If your child is receiving enough insulin for her needs, she will not develop ketoacidosis even if her blood glucose level is high. Eating too much at dinner one night will not cause ketoacidosis if the body has enough insulin to meet its needs.

However, ketoacidosis may occur if your child has very high blood glucose and is vomiting. Illness can cause other hormones such as adrenaline to be released, which then cause the need for extra insulin. These hormones help fight illness, but they also block the action of insulin. This is why you *always* give your child insulin when she is sick—even if she is eating less than usual.

Preventing and Treating Ketoacidosis

You can prevent ketoacidosis by checking the urine for ketones daily (see *Urine Testing*, page 47) and by treating illness and hyperglycemia promptly with your doctor's assistance.

Ketoacidosis must be treated right away, possibly with intravenous (IV) fluids. Call your doctor immediately if your child has any of the symptoms listed in the box below. A trip to the emergency room or a short hospital stay may be necessary.

WHEN TO CALL THE DOCTOR IMMEDIATELY

Check with your child's doctor to learn when you should call. Always call right away if your child has any of the following problems. Your child may be developing ketoacidosis.

■ moderate or high levels of ketones in the urine
■ ketones in the urine for more than one urine test
■ dehydration (symptoms include sunken eyes; dry, cracked lips; dry mouth; skin that remains pinched up after it is pinched)
■ persistent vomiting*
■ any change in alertness or drowsiness
■ labored breathing
■ fruity-smelling breath (an odor like fruity chewing gum or nail polish remover)
■ abdominal pain

If you can't reach the doctor, take the child to an emergency room right away.

*Vomiting can be caused by many illnesses. It is always a potentially serious problem for children with diabetes since it can cause ketoacidosis.

REBOUND (SOMOGYI EFFECT)

Rebound is an abnormal increase in blood glucose that occurs after an episode of low blood glucose. It is called the Somogyi Effect after the doctor who first identified it, Michael Somogyi.

When blood glucose levels fall below normal, the body usually responds by producing extra adrenaline, glucagon, and other hormones that help the body deal with stress. These hormones cause the liver to store glucose and release it into the blood.

This process can help to prevent your child's blood glucose level from dropping too low. Sometimes, however, the adrenaline and glucagon work for hours after blood glucose levels return to normal. This can cause high blood glucose several hours after an episode of low blood glucose.

One clue that this might be happening is a pattern of blood glucose tests that reads low, high, low, high, and so on. Small amounts of ketones in the urine may be another clue. If your child has wide swings in blood glucose levels over the course of a few days, talk to your doctor or diabetes educator.

Reducing the insulin dose often helps fix the bouncing. Although the rebound effect does exist, it has less significance in daily control than previously thought. Some of the high blood glucose that follows a low can be from overtreatment of the low blood sugar with sugary foods or too much food. Seek help from your doctor if your child seems to be experiencing rebound.

DAWN PHENOMENON

People with diabetes frequently experience a rise in blood glucose levels very early in the morning. This increase is called the dawn phenomenon because it occurs at around 4 a.m. due to the release of hormones such as growth hormone.

If your child is consistently awakening in the morning with a high blood glucose, it would be smart to check his blood around midnight, then at 4 a.m. to see what is happening during the night. If the midnight number is okay, but the blood glucose rises from then until morning, more insulin may be needed. The dawn phenomenon can be prevented by increasing the evening NPH or lente insulin dose, or by giving the evening insulin dose at bedtime.

HOW TO HANDLE SICK DAYS

Children with diabetes do not usually get sick more often than other children unless their blood glucose is persistently high. However, children with diabetes need special care when they get sick.

It may be helpful for you and your child's doctors to work out in advance a plan for handling sick days. The plan should include:

▮ phone numbers for reaching a doctor at all times

▮ guidelines for when it is important to call

▮ guidelines for adjusting insulin

▮ guidelines for checking blood glucose and adjusting your child's meal plan

---

HELPFUL HINTS FOR SICK DAYS

Your doctor can give you guidance tailor-made for your child, but the following general hints may be helpful.

▮ Reaching the doctor
Write down phone numbers where you can reach a doctor at all times. Keep these numbers handy.

▮ Insulin
Your child needs insulin every day and may need extra doses on sick days.

▮ Blood and urine testing
Check blood glucose levels at least four times a day. Test urine for ketones frequently. If your child is vomiting or has large amounts of ketones in the urine, test both blood and urine every 2 hours.

▮ Meals
Try small meals and extra snacks. If your child has trouble eating, try special foods. Give your child plenty of fluids to drink.
- If your child is eating, give sugar-free fluids (such as sugar-free sodas or powdered drink mixes).
- If your child is not eating, give fluids that contain sugar and other nutrients (such as nondiet cola, gelatin water (gelatin before it hardens), a Popsicle, clear broth, Gatorade, or Pedialyte).

Giving Insulin During Illness

Your child should always take insulin, even if she is not eating well. Illness and stress can cause a need for more insulin. Children may need higher doses of rapid- or short-acting insulin on sick days to lower blood glucose quickly.

However, if your child is eating poorly or vomiting, she may need less than the usual amount of intermediate- or long-acting insulin. If your child is vomiting or not eating well, call your health care provider for advice on adjusting her insulin dose.

Blood and Urine Testing

It's very important to check blood glucose levels and test urine for ketones more often than usual when your child is sick. The extra tests will help you and the doctor decide how much extra insulin your child needs.

Test blood glucose at least four times a day, and test urine for ketones frequently (several times a day). If your child is vomiting or has large amounts of ketones in her urine, you may need to test both blood and urine every 2 hours. This stepped-up testing schedule should continue until ketones clear, blood glucose is back to normal, and your child feels better.

Eating During Illness

Try to keep your child on her regular meal plan as much as possible. She still needs food to balance her insulin. If your child has trouble eating regular foods, try some of the foods in the box on page 91. Small meals and extra snacks may be better than three big meals.

Encourage your child to drink lots of fluids, especially if she has a fever. It's very easy for a child to become dehydrated during illness. Dehydration robs the body of needed water and nutrients, can disrupt control of diabetes, and may contribute to ketoacidosis.

If your child is eating, it's a good idea for her to drink water or sugar-free sodas, sugar-free powdered drink mixes, or iced tea

EASY FOODS FOR SICK DAYS

These foods are well tolerated by most sick people. They may also be good substitutes when your child has an upset stomach or has trouble eating regular meals (for example, after getting braces).

Fruit Exchange replacements (10 grams of carbohydrate)

1/2 cup (4 oz) regular soft drink with sugar (ginger ale or cola)
1/2 cup (4 oz) fruit juice (orange, grape)
1/2 twin-bar Popsicle
1 fruit exchange (1 orange)
2 Tbsp corn syrup or honey
1/4 cup (2 oz) sweetened gelatin
6 LifeSavers
2 Tbsp (1 oz) Coke syrup

Starch Exchange replacements (15 grams of carbohydrate)

1/2 cup (4 oz) ice cream
1/2 cup (4 oz) cooked cereal
1/4 cup (2 oz) sherbet
1/2 cup sweetened gelatin
2 cups broth-based soup, reconstituted with water
1 cup cream soup
3/4 cup (6 oz) regular soft drink with sugar (ginger ale or cola)
1/4 cup (2 oz) milkshake
1 slice toast
6 soda crackers

Milk Exchange replacements (12 grams of carbohydrate)

5 oz regular soft drink with sugar (ginger ale or cola)
1 cup eggnog
1 cup (8 oz) milk

(which have no calories). If your child is *not* eating, is vomiting, has diarrhea, or has ketones in the urine, she needs fluids that contain carbohydrates and calories.

Recommendations from the American Academy of Pediatrics note that foods with complex carbohydrates such as rice and cereal, lean meat, yogurt, fruit, and vegetables are foods of choice for children who are sick. For diarrhea, your child may need specially formulated products with electrolytes found in your pharmacy. You will need to provide fluids that contain both carbohydrate (sugar) and sodium, such as Sprite, 7-Up, broth, or soup. Glucose tablets, Popsicles, and complex carbohydrates with salt (pretzels or crackers) are treatment for hypoglycemia.

INFECTIONS

If your child's glucose levels are in her target range, she should not get more infections than other children should. However, if she has frequent high blood glucose, she may be more likely to get infections. This is because bacteria grow well in glucose, and bacteria-fighting cells do not work as well in a high-glucose environment. When glucose is high, it's easier to pick up an infection and harder to shake it off.

Yeast Infections

Girls with diabetes may get vaginal infections, especially if they have frequent high blood glucose levels. A fungus called *Candida albicans* causes the most common vaginal infection, often called a yeast infection.

This fungus is normally present in the skin, mouth, intestinal tract, and vagina. When it multiplies abnormally, it can cause an infection. Having a high level of glucose in the blood and taking some kinds of antibiotics can cause an overgrowth of the fungus. Your child's doctor can advise you how to treat a yeast infection. Most of the time it can be easily treated by improving blood glucose control and topical treatment with an over-the-counter anti-fungal cream.

Symptoms of *Candida* infection include itching, burning, and a thick, white or yellow vaginal discharge that can look like cottage cheese. These infections can usually be treated with over-the-counter suppositories or creams. Improving diabetes control can prevent *Candida* infections. Other ways girls with diabetes can protect themselves from *Candida* infections include:

■ Drying the outside vaginal area thoroughly after a shower, bath, or swim. Yeast is less likely to grow in a dry area.

■ Changing out of a wet bathing suit or other wet clothes quickly.

■ Wearing cotton underwear.

■ Avoiding wearing nylon (nonbreathing) clothing, such as spandex tights or shorts, for long periods of time.

■ Avoiding wearing tight jeans if you are prone to infections.

Babies with diabetes can also develop rashes at their diaper area when glucose is high in their urine. If the child is not potty trained and blood glucose is high, careful attention to the diaper area and frequent changing is important. If a diaper rash persists, your doctor can recommend a cream or ointment.

TAKING CARE OF TEETH AND GUMS

Children with diabetes usually do not have more dental problems than other children. They probably eat less candy and sugar than other children do, so they should have a lower risk of cavities.

However, *gingivitis* (inflammation of the gums) can be a long-term complication of diabetes. Gingivitis can lead to *periodontitis*, a more severe gum disease in which bone is lost and spaces develop between the gums and the teeth. Following healthy dental practices in childhood may prevent dental problems later on.

It's a good idea to brush teeth for a full 2 minutes twice a day and preferable to do it after every meal. If you treat low blood glucose with sweets at night, try to have your child brush her teeth afterward, or try to wash the sweet food down with water to rinse away sugar between the teeth. Take your child for regular dental checkups. If your child has red, swollen gums or any other dental problem, call your dentist immediately.

If your child needs to have extensive work or dental surgery, ask your dentist to call your doctor so that the child's insulin dose can be adjusted on the day of the procedure and for a few days afterward. If your child's eating habits change after having dental surgery or getting braces, insulin will need to be adjusted. Stay in touch with your doctor or diabetes educator when your child is having dental work done.

THYROID DISEASE

The thyroid is a gland located in the neck. Hormones made by the thyroid gland help to control the way the body works (the metabolism).

The body can sometimes attack and destroy the beta cells that make insulin. This is called an *autoimmune attack*. Other antibodies can attack and destroy the thyroid gland, causing thyroid disease. The reasons why autoimmune attacks occur are not known.

People who already have one autoimmune disease (diabetes) are at increased risk of developing another one. Therefore, people with type 1 diabetes are more likely than other people to develop thyroid disease.

There are two kinds of thyroid disease. *Hyperthyroidism* occurs when the thyroid gland makes too much of a hormone called thyroxine. This disease is uncommon in children with diabetes. *Hypothyroidism* occurs when the thyroid does not make enough thyroxine. This disease is more common in children with diabetes than in other children.

When the thyroid gland is damaged by an autoimmune attack, it may get bigger and try to go on making normal amounts of thyroxine. This can cause a swelling in the front part of the neck called a *goiter*. In time, the thyroid may no longer make normal amounts of thyroxine and symptoms of hypothyroidism appear. These symptoms include:

▌ weight gain
▌ feeling tired or cold
▌ dry skin or hair loss

■ constipation

■ irregular menstrual periods

If hypothyroidism is not treated it can affect a child's growth. Your child's doctor can check for hypothyroidism by feeling her thyroid gland and checking the level of thyroxine in the blood. This level should be checked at least once a year. Thyroid disease is easily treated with a pill containing thyroxine, the hormone that the thyroid gland is no longer making.

COMPLICATIONS OF DIABETES

People who have diabetes for a long time may get other diseases that are caused by diabetes. These other diseases are complications of diabetes. It is rare for children to have complications. However, your child may be at risk for complications when she has had diabetes for 15 years or more.

Complications of diabetes can include blood vessel problems that lead to kidney disease, heart disease, eye disease, and nerve disease. In the Diabetes Control and Complications Trial (DCCT), doctors found that maintaining near-normal blood glucose levels ("tight control") prevented or postponed many complications of diabetes. (See page 11.)

Achieving tight control takes time, money, and energy. But the DCCT results demonstrate that the effort involved is worthwhile and give people with diabetes more hope for a healthy future.

Although complications of diabetes are rare in childhood, teaching your child healthy habits while she is young can help to prevent or reduce complications when she becomes an adult. For example, learning to keep feet clean and telling you when they are bruised or cut will be important later in life to reduce the risk of foot problems.

When your child is 12 years old and has had diabetes for 5 years, she should start seeing an *eye specialist* once a year for a screening. This can be an *ophthalmologist* (a doctor who specializes in treating eye diseases) or an *optometrist* trained to perform dilated eye exams, not an *optician* who fits glasses. In the unlikely event that eye disease is found, she should be seen by an ophthalmologist.

Your doctor should periodically check for protein in your child's urine (a sign of kidney disease) and her blood pressure and cholesterol levels.

Children and teens need to be aware that complications of diabetes do happen, and that they can prevent them. But trying to frighten youngsters into changing their behavior by threatening future complications has not been shown to be effective in most cases.

Seventeen-year-old Susan had always had difficulty keeping her blood glucose in the target range. A well-meaning uncle tried to scare her: "Susan, you'll go blind like your grandmother." But instead of improving her diabetes care in response to this threat, Susan decided that if she was going to go blind there was no point in making an effort to maintain good glucose control. A better approach would have been to talk with Susan openly about her problems with diabetes care, help her understand that controlling blood glucose levels really can prevent complications once thought inevitable, and support her efforts to reach her goals.

If your child is worried about getting complications in the future, it may help to have a talk with her doctor. Your child may also benefit from counseling to help her adjust to living with diabetes. Open discussion of fears can help to make them easier to bear.

As the parent of a child with diabetes, you too may have fears about the future. Feel free to discuss these fears with your health care provider. Your providers may be able to recommend a counselor who can help you to deal with these worries. Seeking help from a counselor is never a sign of weakness. On the contrary, it's a sign that you want to make life with diabetes the best it can be.

IF YOUR CHILD HAS TYPE 2 DIABETES

Although type 2 diabetes mostly happens in adults, it can occur in children. In the past, it was rare for children or adolescents to get type 2 diabetes. Recently, however, there has been an increase of type 2 diabetes in children throughout the world. Scientists believe this is caused by changes in society as children eat more fast foods, watch more TV, and play endless video and computer games. Today's children are heavier and more sedentary.

The signs and symptoms of type 2 in children are usually the same as the signs for type 1 diabetes (see page 4). Most adolescents with type 2 diabetes are overweight, eat a high-calorie diet, and don't get much exercise.

In type 2 diabetes, the pancreas makes insulin. However, the body cells can't use the insulin that is circulating. This is called *insulin resistance*. Insulin resistance means body cells can't get the glucose they need from the bloodstream. Insulin resistance gets worse with weight gain, and is improved by weight loss and exercise.

There are several ways to take care of type 2 diabetes. Many adolescents with type 2 diabetes need to take insulin by injection. The doctor will decide which kinds of insulin are best and how often they need to be taken. Often adolescents with type 2 diabetes can be taken off insulin if blood glucose levels are lowered and they are successful in losing some weight or increasing their activity level.

Controlling diabetes with pills alone or insulin plus pills is another treatment option for those with type 2 diabetes. Since a main problem is obesity, the main treatment is diet and exercise. A loss of excess body fat and improvement in exercise habits are the best way to treat insulin resistance. Unfortunately, making these lifestyle changes can be challenging. If your child has type 2 diabetes, you and your child should work closely with the diabetes team, especially the dietitian.

Since type 2 diabetes in children is a new problem, scientists are still studying which diabetes medications and regimens might be most effective. The use of pills in this age group is based on what we know from treating adults.

To find out what works best (insulin and/or pills) in controlling your child's blood sugars, your child will need to test her blood glucose. The doctor can tell when she will need to test.

It will also be important for your child to have her blood tested for HbA_{1c} levels (see page 50).

Just like the child with type 1 diabetes, the child with type 2 diabetes is also at risk for getting infections and complications later. In most cases, serious diabetes complications are not inevitable and can be prevented. This is why keeping blood sugars as close to normal as possible is so important.

As Your Child Grows Up

Growing up brings special challenges and rewards for both children and parents. Growing up with diabetes is an additional challenge, and growing up healthy brings special rewards, not only for your child but also for you.

All parents worry about their children, but it's natural for you to worry a little more about your child with diabetes. By presenting an overview of situations you may encounter as your child grows up, this chapter may help you to worry a bit less.

WHEN BABY HAS DIABETES

With good medical care, babies with diabetes grow and develop into healthy, active children. Your doctor and other health care providers can help you to adjust insulin and food intake so your infant will grow and gain weight normally. You can expect your baby to roll over, sit up, crawl, and talk the same time as other babies.

If your baby is hospitalized, you may find that he briefly loses some of the skills he had developed or goes back to acting the way he did at a younger age. For example, an infant who drank from a cup may insist on a bottle for a while after coming home from the hospital. This behavior is not caused by diabetes. Any child who undergoes a stressful experience like being hospitalized may cope by seeking comfort in familiar things like a pacifier. Once your baby settles down at home again, he will soon regain any lost skills and continue to develop normally.

How Can I Tell If My Baby Has Low Blood Glucose?

Parents are usually most worried about low blood glucose in infancy because babies can't tell their parents that they feel strange. You will need to learn to look for signs like these that tell you your baby's glucose is low:

- sweating
- pale skin
- irritability
- tiredness
- shaking
- crying
- enlarged pupils
- restlessness at night
- bluish color around the lips

Regular blood glucose tests are very important in babies. Your doctor or nurse educator can help you learn to do these tests. Blood may be taken from heels, toes, or earlobes if little fingers

---

TESTING A WET DIAPER FOR URINE GLUCOSE

1. Many brands of disposable diapers contain silica gel to retain moisture and keep baby dry (call the manufacturer to find out). If the diapers you use contain silica gel, place a diaper liner or a few cotton balls inside your baby's diaper.
2. Pull some of the wet stuffing out of the diaper liner and push it into an empty syringe.
3. Push in the syringe plunger to squeeze out a drop of urine.
4. Place the drop of urine on a test strip and "read" the strip.

---

become tender from too many fingersticks. See the box on page 99 for a way to test a baby's wet diaper for urine glucose.

It is always a good idea to treat your baby if you are unsure whether he is having a low. *When in doubt, treat.*

**TREATING A BABY FOR
LOW BLOOD GLUCOSE**

1. Give the baby a sugary drink (such as apple juice, sugar water, or glucose gel). This should have an effect within 20 minutes.
2. Follow with formula or milk (which provides complex carbohydrate and protein). If the baby is eating solids, you may give cereal, vegetables, or meat instead of milk.
3. If the baby won't eat or if symptoms don't improve, give a glucagon injection and call your doctor. Make sure you already have instructions from your doctor on how much glucagon to give your baby. Half the usual dose of glucagon (0.5 mg) is often suggested for infants.

Illnesses in Infancy

Infants with diabetes don't get infections, colds, or diarrhea more than other babies. If your baby with diabetes does get sick, be sure to follow your doctor's sick-day guidelines.

Sick-day guidelines for babies are the same as those for older children (see *How to Handle Sick Days*, page 88). However, a baby can become very sick more quickly than an older child can because an infant becomes dehydrated faster. Symptoms of dehydration include:

▌ sunken eyes
▌ dry, cracked lips
▌ dry mouth
▌ skin that remains pinched up after being pinched

Because of the risk of dehydration, make sure your baby continues to take in fluids when he is sick and call your doctor immediately. It's very important to check for ketones frequently when your baby is sick.

Babies with diabetes who have diarrhea should be treated in the same way that any other child with diarrhea would be treated. Give liquids with electrolytes or foods that contain both carbohydrate and sodium.

Your baby may need less insulin when he has diarrhea or another illness that causes him to eat less than usual. Talk to your doctor or diabetes educator about how to adjust insulin during illness.

IF YOUR BABY IS VOMITING OR HAS DIARRHEA

1. **Call the doctor right away.**
2. Begin to give the baby small amounts of sugary fluids, such as apple juice, sugar water, gelatin water (gelatin before it hardens), Pedialyte, or other preparations from the pharmacy made for this purpose.

If Your Baby Won't Eat

All babies go through stages when they won't eat. However, babies with diabetes need food to balance their insulin. If your baby won't eat, and isn't yet on solid food, you can try offering other fluids (like juice, sugar water, or Pedialyte). If the baby is on solids, try offering a different food, or else try fluids.

If your baby refuses both solids and fluids, wait 10 minutes and try again. Offering small amounts frequently may be helpful. It's never a good idea to force your infant to eat. You may have to settle for feeding the baby any foods (or fluids) that he likes, such as ice cream, pudding, tapioca, or cookies. For a baby with diabetes, this is always preferable to no food.

Coping When Your Baby Has Diabetes

Caring for an infant with diabetes can be difficult and stressful. It's natural for parents to worry about their baby having low blood glucose or not eating or about giving the baby insulin injections.

For your own mental well-being, it's important that you be able to take a break from caring for your baby with diabetes for an afternoon, an evening, or a weekend. If you and your spouse are sharing the care, you need uninterrupted time together. Find a person you trust—for example, a friend, an aunt, a grandparent, or a kindly neighbor—who can care for your baby while you take a break. This caregiver will need general training in diabetes care and an understanding of your baby's care routine. Some parents find it helps their peace of mind to use a pager or cell phone when they are away, so that the caregiver can keep in touch with them.

Your doctor, dietitian, diabetes educator, or social worker may be able to suggest additional sources of support when you become very worried or stressed. Asking for help is never a sign of weakness. You have a lot to do and cope with. (See *Asking for Help*, page 140.)

YOUR PRESCHOOLER WITH DIABETES

Parents of a preschooler with diabetes may have the same feelings of anxiety and helplessness that parents of infants have. Low blood glucose can still be a big worry. You still need to be on the lookout for signs of low blood glucose (see pages 7 and 78–79) because your child can't always tell you how he is feeling. Frequent blood glucose checks are a good way to reassure yourself that your child is all right.

How Can I Help My Child to Accept Fingersticks and Insulin Injections?

Insulin injections and regular blood glucose tests are very important to your child's diabetes care. But the needles and fingersticks can be frightening to a preschooler. The invasion of his body may be especially threatening to a child at this age.

It may help to say to your child: "Yes, I know this pinches and I'm sorry," and "You're being very brave." Let the child choose which finger to use for the fingerstick or where to give the insulin injection. Feeling that he has some control over the situation may help to ease the child's anxiety. An adhesive bandage to cover the wound and a hug or a kiss when it's over may be all it takes to smooth things out.

You may want to try using stickers or star charts as incentives to help your child accept fingersticks and injections. Explain that every time he has a fingerstick or an injection, he will earn a star or sticker. When he has 20 or 25 stars, he can plan a special treat like a trip to the zoo or the library.

Young children may try to delay fingersticks and injections. They'll say, "Wait just one more minute and I'll be ready." But one minute soon becomes 15 and the child is late for preschool. One solution to this problem is to use a cooking timer. Set the timer for 10 minutes and explain that if the child has the fingerstick or injection before the bell rings, he will earn a star. But if the procedure isn't done when the bell rings, he won't get a reward.

Praise your child for being brave and holding still while you give the injection. Try not to scold him for moving during the fingerstick or for being late for an injection.

At times, however, even praise and the offer of rewards may not help. Your child just won't cooperate. Preschoolers may find it hard to understand why they need injections, especially if they don't feel sick.

If this happens, you may have to hold the child or get someone to help you give the injection. This is never pleasant, but your child needs to get insulin regularly. Afterward, it may be helpful to hug your child and explain that you have to give the injections "to keep you well."

Children often express their frustrations and worries through play. Having your preschooler give an injection to a favorite doll or stuffed animal may help him express his fears.

Four-year-old Larry was terrified of getting his insulin injections. His mother reported that he avoided going to bed at night because he associated waking up in the morning with getting an injection. He woke up during the night with nightmares about the injection. Every morning his parents chased him through the house to give him his insulin.

One day, Larry's mother began including his favorite stuffed animal in the procedure. Before giving Larry his insulin, she went through the entire routine with the toy, including placing a Band-Aid over the injection site. Finally, Larry began giving his "diabetic bunny" the injection. Through play, he was able to express feelings that he couldn't express in words. Eventually, he got over his fear of injections.

How Can I Get My Child to Eat Regularly?

Getting a youngster with diabetes to eat properly can be just as challenging as giving fingersticks and insulin injections. Young children often try to take control at mealtimes.

The most effective way of handling a child who fusses at meals may be to not make an issue of eating or not eating. If the child rejects a meal, offer something else. If that's rejected, try offering orange juice or a piece of fruit. Give rapid-acting insulin based on what your child actually eats. The meal can be offered again later. Watch carefully for signs of low blood glucose if your child is going through a fussy eating phase.

Don't let your child prolong meals so that breakfast, snack, and lunch all seem to run together. Allow a certain amount of time for meals. When the time is up, the meal is over. Without this kind of discipline, your child will be nibbling constantly and his blood glucose will always be out of control.

When your child is not eating well, try not to nag or physically force him to eat. Usually, this kind of pressure will only increase the child's resistance. Instead, try providing positive rewards for behavior you want to encourage. Sometimes when children are not in the mood for eating an entire meal, they may be willing to drink something. A carbohydrate-containing beverage, such as milk or flavored milk, may help prevent low blood glucose later on.

It's common for children to want to eat nothing but peanut butter sandwiches for days on end and then to suddenly switch to wanting nothing but hot dogs. As long as the current favorite food is low in fat and sugar, it's okay to let your child eat it as many days in a row as he wants.

Two-year-old Laura was the youngest of 3 children. School mornings for the family were hectic. Laura got her insulin injection and her breakfast while her mother was busy getting the older children ready for the school bus. Although Laura liked her breakfast cereal, she never finished eating it. Because she had not eaten enough food, Laura always had low blood glucose before lunch. After talking with the diabetes educator about this, Laura's mother changed the family's morning routine. Now she waits until the older children have left for school before giving Laura her insulin injection. Then she makes sure that Laura eats her breakfast and has a midmorning snack to prevent low blood glucose.

What If My Child Needs to Be Hospitalized?

Being hospitalized for newly diagnosed diabetes can be very stressful for a child. It can be scary and confusing. The child may think that having diabetes or being in the hospital is a punishment for being bad. It's important to try to reassure your child that none of these things is his fault.

Your child may be anxious or afraid about being away from home. It helps if you can stay with your child while he is in the hospital. Most children's units will let parents stay with their children. If you can't stay, it's important to try to tell your child why, and perhaps find a substitute. Be honest about when you will be back. Leaving the child's favorite toy or blanket can help to ease his anxiety. Pictures or a parent's possession (like a scarf or a handkerchief) are another good reminder of home and family.

For many parents, the period of their child's hospitalization is a time to learn (in a safe environment) as much as they can about their new responsibilities as the parents of a child with diabetes. If your child is not hospitalized when he is diagnosed, you may be able to attend an outpatient program about diabetes care for parents. In either case, diabetes educators will provide help and advice as you learn to give insulin injections and do blood tests.

Daycare and Preschool

When you decide to send your young child to preschool or daycare, the decision of where to go is sometimes difficult. Although any setting that receives any kind of federal funding cannot discriminate about taking a child with a chronic illness or disability, liability concerns, staffing issues, and insurance policies often dictate whether or not a child is accepted into a daycare facility. You will be most concerned about your child's safety, and it is necessary that you ensure that all staff members are informed and knowledgeable about diabetes and your child's individual care plan. You'll want to pay special attention to educating the staff about hypoglycemia: how to recognize the symptoms and provide proper treatment.

This will involve carefully screening and selecting a daycare facility, educating the staff, putting together a diabetes care plan that includes courses of action based on blood glucose readings (see the sample plan on pages 107–108), and keeping in close communication with the staff. Usually after the staff members understand the issues of diabetes and become comfortable with how to care for your child, they will welcome him.

SAMPLE DIABETES CARE PLAN

Guidelines for Caring for

1. When to do a blood glucose check

a. She says, "I'm low," especially if during or after exercise.

b. If she has symptoms of low blood glucose, including:
- irritability
- erratic responses to questions
- sleepiness

2. What to do based on your child's blood sugar reading
(this is an example only and should be adapted to your own child's needs)

60 or Under Give two glucose tablets, followed immediately by food containing 30 grams of carbohydrates. If she doesn't respond or blood glucose levels do not rise within 10 minutes, telephone

(mother)   at   or

(father)   at

for further instructions.

61 to 100 Give one glucose tablet. If a meal or snack is within 30 minutes, she can wait. Otherwise, give her a snack including carbohydrates and protein, such as cheese crackers with peanut butter or cookies and milk.

101 to 140 She is fine. If exercise is planned before a meal or snack, she must have a snack before participating. This includes recess.

141 to 300 She's fine, but higher than we'd like. No action is necessary.

(continued)

Over 240 Her blood glucose is too high. She must be given water or other non-caloric fluids. Allow bathroom use, if needed.

She needs to check her urine for ketones. If ketones are present, the parents or diabetes team should be called for advice. If moderate to large amounts of ketones are present, she may need emergency help immediately.

3. **When giving glucose, the following are roughly equivalent:**
   - Four ounces of fruit juice
   - 1/2 to 1 cup of milk
   - Two glucose tablets
   - One tube of Cake Mate cake decorating gel. If unable to swallow, place between the cheek and gums.
   - One-half can of soda (regular, NOT diet)
   - Two tablespoons of raisins
   - 6 jellybeans
   - 10 gumdrops
   - 5 to 7 lifesavers

Chocolate candy should not be used unless there is no other sugar source available. The fats in chocolate slow the absorption of sugar and provide too many calories and too much cholesterol.

If the blood sugar remains low despite treatment and the student is not thinking clearly, the parents or diabetes care team should be called for advice.

Following an episode of hypoglycemia (low blood glucose), it can take several hours to fully recover. The student can return to the classroom, but may not perform at optimal levels.

THE SCHOOL-AGE YEARS

Children ages 6 to 12 usually have a lot of energy and are eager to learn and do things. They have a vivid imagination, a conscience, and the ability to share and cooperate. They display their energy in horseplay, teasing, schoolwork, games, and fantasy. They have an increasing desire for independence, but they still want their parents' protection and authority.

Starting school or moving on to middle school is a new challenge that may cause a child with diabetes to feel insecure at times. He is meeting a lot of new people and facing new demands such as increased homework and competitive school sports. He may become anxious because his parents aren't always with him.

Parents, in turn, may try to overprotect a child with diabetes. When the child starts going to school, it may be the first time the parent has been separated from the child.

For these reasons, it may be hard for a child with diabetes to be as independent as other children his age. Balancing a child's needs for independence and protection is hard. Yet you help your child most by encouraging him to lead as normal a life as possible while still taking good care of his diabetes.

If you have concerns about how to balance your child's needs for independence and protection, you may want to discuss your feelings with your doctor or diabetes educator. School-age children are often ready to do more of their diabetes care than their parents think they can handle. However, they generally feel more secure when a parent or another adult, such as the school nurse or a teacher, supervises and supports their diabetes care efforts.

How to Handle Troublesome Periods

As children begin to develop their own identities and separate from their parents, they may go through periods of struggle against adults. This is a normal part of growing up, but the struggle may be harder for a child with diabetes who has to take insulin, check glucose and urine all the time, and follow a meal plan.

There are no easy solutions. It may help to talk with your child about his concerns. Talking over his feelings about having diabetes can help to ease his tension, and also help you understand what he is going through. Encourage other family members to talk to your child and offer their support. Sometimes your child with diabetes will benefit from talking with another adult, such as a favorite teacher, school counselor, doctor, nurse, social worker, or minister.

Learning about diabetes and taking on self-care tasks may help your child to come to terms with having diabetes. Often when children are diagnosed with diabetes very young, they never learn basic information about the disease. Understanding how the disease works and why they need to take insulin, check their blood glucose, and so on can help children to accept having diabetes. As your child grows and develops, both you and he will need continuing education about diabetes.

Realize that it can take years for a child or adult to come to terms with having diabetes. Be patient and loving with your child as he learns to handle this difficult challenge.

Diabetes and Your Child's Friends

When children start school, their relationships with their friends become very important to them. Your child's attitude about diabetes can influence his friends' attitudes. If your child accepts diabetes positively, it's likely that his friends will do the same. You can help your child to develop a positive attitude by demonstrating your love, support, and understanding.

Your child's friends may be fearful because they lack information about diabetes. Encourage your child to be open about the disease with his friends. However, a child's willingness to be open about diabetes will depend on his personality. Sometimes a child with diabetes feels sensitive about being different from his friends because he has to take insulin, test blood glucose, and follow a meal plan.

Some children have checked their blood glucose or given themselves an insulin injection for show-and-tell. Older children have presented science projects on diabetes and its care. However, a child who is sensitive or shy about having diabetes may not wish to draw attention to himself in this way. Understanding your child's personality will help you to handle these situations in the way that works best for him.

Communicating with Your Child's School and Teachers

Your child's teachers, the school nurse, and the principal of your child's school all need to know about his diabetes.

When your child starts school, changes schools, or has a new teacher, it's a good idea for parents to ask for a conference meeting with all of these people. This way, everyone hears the same information at the same time and their questions can be answered. Having a written plan that includes important phone numbers is also helpful. Ask the school staff to inform you whenever there is a change to the school schedule that affects your child's meal times or exercise routine, so you can plan ahead.

You can get pamphlets for school staff from your local chapter of the American Diabetes Association, or from www.diabetes.org (use the search function to find "Children with Diabetes: Information for Teachers and Child-Care Providers"). These brochures explain diabetes and how to treat low and high blood glucose. This kind of information will help school staff to feel more secure when dealing with your child.

The School's Legal Responsibilities Regarding Your Child with Diabetes

The level of health care assistance available at your child's school will vary. Few schools today employ a full-time school nurse. Often one school nurse covers an entire school district and in some states the role of the school nurse may no longer exist.

Schools often rely on the school secretary or a health aide to provide emergency health care.

Under federal law, diabetes is considered a disability, and it is illegal for schools to discriminate in any way against a person with a disability. Federal law also requires that anyone with a disability have full access to public programs, which include the public schools. In addition, federal law entitles children with diabetes to special education services if they need them.

When a school is notified that a child has diabetes, it must do an evaluation of the child's special needs. This might require obtaining medical information from the child's doctor or health care team. The school must prepare a plan that outlines how the child's special health care needs will be met so that he has an equal opportunity to take part in all school programs.

The school must consult you, the child's parent, about the plan, and it cannot alter the plan without your consent. A school staff member must be designated to be responsible for implementing the plan, and other school staff must know what the plan requires them to do. The plan should be updated every year.

You will find that most schools are very cooperative and want to help. If, however, your child is having problems and the school is not supportive, you will need to step in. Most laws that protect schoolchildren with diabetes have been made because of parents who insisted on having a safe and healthy setting for their children. If you have problems or feel that your child is not being treated fairly, contact the American Diabetes Association's Government Relations Division for help. Your local ADA chapter can help guide you.

Checking Blood Glucose at School

Parents and school personnel should meet at the beginning of each school year to put together an individualized diabetes care plan for your child. This should include meals, snacks, target blood glucose levels, schedules, how to handle exercise, symptoms of high and low blood glucose, when and where to test, and a plan for hypoglycemia. Most children in schools should be testing blood glucose before lunch, and before taking part in a strenuous sport like basketball or football.

Decide with school staff and your child where the best place is to test. Find out which school staff member is responsible for helping your child to do a blood test, and ask him or her to record the test result. This will help you to monitor patterns in your child's glucose levels.

Your child may feel uncomfortable about doing blood tests at school, or it may really disrupt his school routine to have to do the tests. If this is the case, ask your diabetes educator for advice about how often testing is necessary and how to fit it in during a busy school day.

What If My Child Has Low Blood Glucose at School?

Your child's teachers and other school staff, such as the secretary, health aide, or school nurse (if there is one) need to know the signs of low blood glucose (see pages 7 and 78–79). Subtle signs can be missed unless the school staff is well informed. For example, these behaviors may be signs of undetected low blood glucose:

■ midmorning sleepiness
■ lack of attention in class just before lunch or in midafternoon
■ complaints of a headache after gym class

Most elementary school teachers can treat your child in the classroom by giving him a glucose tablet and crackers to eat (if he is not treating the episode on his own).

Be sure to stress that your child should not be sent to the nurse's office alone. A friend should go along in case low blood glucose causes your child to become dizzy or confused.

It's a good idea to give a supply of sugar cubes, glucose tablets, crackers, or small juice boxes to your child's teacher, as well as to your child, for emergencies. You may want the gym teacher to have a supply as well.

Your child's teachers should also know how to give a glucagon injection. However, many school districts do not allow school personnel to give glucagon injections. Find out what your school district's policy is when you meet with your school's staff.

Some children may feel anxious about low blood glucose and ask to leave the classroom a lot. They may not have learned to tell the difference between feeling anxious and the symptoms of low blood glucose. Alternatively, they may be seeking attention or trying to get out of class. The fastest way to stop this behavior is to ask for a blood glucose test whenever the child wishes to leave the room. If blood glucose isn't low, the child should stay in class.

Handling Snacks at School

Your child may need to eat one or more snacks during the school day. You may decide to send a supply of snacks to be kept at the school or to pack snacks daily with the child's lunch.

Usually your child should also eat a snack before gym class. If gym is right after a meal, the snack should be eaten after the class rather than before. Crackers with peanut butter or cheese, pretzels, apples, or small cans of juice are ideal snacks.

Some teachers have used classroom snack time to teach children about healthy eating. Instead of cookies and milk, they may serve popcorn or a cereal mix. This not only helps the child with diabetes to feel like one of the gang, but it also teaches healthy eating habits to the other children.

What If My Child Has High Blood Glucose at School?

It's important to explain to the staff of your child's school the signs of high blood glucose (see page 5). It may be helpful to also explain that when your child's blood glucose is running a bit high, he may need to make extra trips to the bathroom or the water fountain.

> John had just started middle school and learned that lunch was served at 10:15 a.m. Because he took his insulin at 8 a.m., 10:15 was early to be having lunch. John wanted to eat lunch with his classmates, but he worried that he might have low blood glucose in the afternoon because his next scheduled snack wasn't until 3 p.m. He solved the problem by adding a small snack at 1 p.m., which he ate on his way to math class. The extra snack prevented him from having low blood glucose in the afternoon. This solution enabled John to eat with his friends and still maintain good blood glucose control.

You may want to ask your child's teacher or the school nurse to tell you when your child has signs of high blood glucose. These signs may indicate that your child's insulin dosage needs to be adjusted.

School Lunches and Parties

Many schools make lunch menus available ahead of time, giving you and your child a chance to plan. (See *How Can I Help My Child to Accept Meal Planning?* page 64.)

When you talk with the staff at your child's school, you may want to mention that your child tries to avoid eating fatty foods and sweets. This will help them to be sensitive to your child's needs at special events or parties. But teachers and other school staff should not be expected to keep an eye on what your child eats every day.

School parties can be hard on children with diabetes. Your child will want to eat the same party food that the other children are eating. Ask the teacher to let you know when a party is planned and suggest that he or she also speak to the parents of the child who is having the party. Some teachers will encourage all parents to bring party foods that all the children can eat. If you have time and know ahead what's happening in school, you might send in a bag of air-popped popcorn or pretzels so the children have some low-fat options during the party. (See *Holidays and Parties*, page 67.)

> The cafeteria staff at 10-year-old Drew's school knew about his diabetes and wanted to be helpful. Every day when Drew bought his lunch, a cafeteria aide would check his tray to make sure he selected a health lunch. Drew, embarrassed by this, stopped eating his lunch. As a result, he started having low blood glucose in the early afternoon. When Drew's mother found out what was happening, she arranged to meet with the school staff, thanked the cafeteria aides, but asked them not to check on Drew's food choices. Drew was then able to eat his lunch without embarrassment.

Will My Child Have to Miss a Lot of School?

Your child with diabetes should not have to miss school more than other children. Frequent absences from school may be a signal that your child's diabetes is not being controlled as well as it could be.

Frequent absences may also be a warning sign that your child is struggling emotionally. Sometimes a child may try to use diabetes as an excuse to avoid going to school. If this happens, you may want to seek advice from a doctor, social worker, school counselor, psychologist, or psychiatrist. (See *Asking for Help*, page 140.)

SHOULD I SEND MY CHILD TO DIABETES CAMP?

Going to camp can be a good experience for any child. Camps geared to children with diabetes make sure that the experience is safe and healthy. Most diabetes camps have these goals:

■ giving children the opportunity to meet other children who have diabetes

■ helping children to be more self-sufficient by teaching them about diabetes and self-care

Each diabetes camp has its own way of teaching children about diabetes. Some camps use schoolroom-type lectures. Others have a much more informal structure.

Going to camp seems to help most children with diabetes. They learn more about their condition and often learn to give their own insulin injections for the first time. At camp, children with diabetes meet many other children who share the same problems. After leaving camp, children often become pen pals and continue to share their feelings and fears.

Camp can provide an opportunity for children to learn independence and assume self-care tasks. Parents can feel comfortable knowing that the camp staff is trained to handle problems related to diabetes.

For a complete list of camps for children with diabetes, contact your local chapter of the American Diabetes Association (in the white pages of the phone book). The American Diabetes Association can also give you information about weekend trips for teens, family camps, and year-round activities.

DIABETES AND YOUR CHILD'S HEIGHT AND WEIGHT

Children, especially teenagers, are often very concerned about their appearance and may want to know how diabetes can affect it. Children with diabetes do not look any different from other children.

However, if diabetes is not well cared for, it may affect a child's height and weight. Thyroid disease may also cause growth problems (see page 93). Your child's doctor should monitor his height and weight carefully.

Sudden weight loss can be a sign of uncontrolled diabetes. When the body isn't making enough insulin, it breaks down fat to obtain energy and eliminates more water than usual, causing weight to drop. Once your child's blood glucose levels are brought under control, he should regain the lost weight.

If Your Child Wants to Lose Weight

Losing weight can be hard for a plump child or teen with diabetes because he must eat regularly to cover insulin. A child with diabetes cannot go on a crash diet.

Sometimes teenagers with diabetes decide that losing weight is more important than controlling blood glucose levels. If a teen skips meals or cuts calories without reducing insulin, he can end up with severe low blood glucose. Teens may also try to lose weight by cutting down on insulin, which can cause severe high blood glucose.

If a child with diabetes wants to lose weight, it is best to get help from a doctor and/or a dietitian. Weight loss through a low-calorie diet that limits fat intake, provides the right nutrients, and controls blood glucose levels may take longer, but it will be safer.

When a lower-calorie diet is recommended, it's important to reduce insulin. Getting more exercise is often the most helpful weight-loss strategy.

Fad diets and diet pills are very popular, especially among teenage girls. However, fad diets can be harmful because they may not provide enough nutrients. In people with diabetes, a fad diet can upset blood glucose control.

Over-the-counter diet pills may work for a short time, but many people soon regain weight. Because diet pills can cause dizziness, nervousness, anxiety, sleeplessness, and other side effects, they are generally not recommended for children and teens.

Joining a weight-loss program can be helpful. Teens, especially, seem to do better at weight loss in a group with other teens.

BROTHERS AND SISTERS

Siblings can be a great asset to a child with diabetes. Because brothers and sisters usually know each other well and notice unusual behavior, a sibling may be the first to pick up signs of low blood glucose.

How Will Having a Child with Diabetes Affect My Other Children?

Because a youngster with diabetes gets a lot of attention, brothers and sisters may sometimes feel anxious or neglected. Seeing their brother or sister with low blood glucose can be frightening, especially for younger siblings, who may fear that the child with diabetes will die. Brothers and sisters may think that their angry feelings or bad thoughts caused their sibling to get sick.

Amy, a teenager with newly diagnosed diabetes, was having a hard time accepting her insulin injections. Every morning she created a scene by refusing her insulin. The whole family's attention was on her, including that of her adoring 3-year-old brother. No one realized how her scenes were affecting him until one morning he began crying and begged his mother to give him the injection instead. When Amy realized that her behavior was hurting her brother, she calmed down and accepted the shots.

It is important to talk these fears over with children and reassure them that they did not cause their sibling's diabetes. Once they are about 5 or 6, children can take part in educational sessions about diabetes and can be encouraged to help with the care of their sibling with diabetes.

Brothers and sisters may be afraid of getting diabetes themselves. The chance that this will happen is very slim. Studies show that about 5 out of every 100 siblings of a child with diabetes may get diabetes by age 30.

How Brothers and Sisters Can Help

Brothers and sisters can be taught the signs and symptoms of low blood glucose and can help parents watch for these signs in the child with diabetes. For example, a sibling who shares a bedroom with the child with diabetes can be taught to alert parents when the child has nightmares or sleeps restlessly. Siblings who are mature enough can help with blood testing or with giving insulin injections.

But brothers and sisters are not substitute parents. Although they may be very willing to help when their sibling with diabetes needs them, they should not be forced to assume the burden of caring for their sibling.

Ten-year-old Matt, who has diabetes, was on the same soccer team as his brother Peter, 12. If Matt experienced low blood glucose during an active game, the coach always asked Peter to sit out of the game while Matt treated himself. This made Peter angry. He was willing to help if his brother needed him but didn't like being forced to sit out of the game because of Matt. When he told his father what was happening, his father asked the coach not to make Peter leave the game to help Matt.

Fourteen-year-old Anne and her 11-year-old sister Wendy played on a softball team together. One day during a game Anne noticed that Wendy was stumbling a lot and throwing the ball poorly. She gave her sister sugar cubes and crackers. Wendy went on to hit a winning home run.

Planning Meals for the Family

It's a good idea for the whole family to eat the same meals instead of serving a separate meal for the child with diabetes. This helps the child with diabetes to feel part of the family. Other family members benefit by learning healthy eating habits. When siblings understand the dietary needs of the child with diabetes, they can help him to select healthy foods.

Some parents may feel that they are punishing their other children by not having sweets in the house. They buy foods for the other children that the child with diabetes can't eat. This is very hard on the child with diabetes, who may not have enough self-control to refuse to eat candy or other treats. As one teenage girl remarked, "When cookies are sitting there, it's hard not to want them."

All children need to know that following a healthy meal plan is not a punishment, but a lifelong habit that will help them to stay well and keep them from being fat or getting cavities. The meal plan for your child with diabetes can be flexible enough to include occasional sweet treats (see page 58). Parents may also suggest to their other children that they eat sweets occasionally when they are out with their friends instead of at home.

> Nine-year-old Keisha saw her two teenage brothers eating cookies and potato chips every day—foods that Keisha wasn't allowed to eat because she had diabetes. But when her parents weren't watching, Keisha would help herself to the cookies and chips. When her mother found out, she became upset with Keisha. Keisha told her mother how sad she felt when she saw the boys eating snacks that she wasn't allowed to have. A family meeting was arranged, and Keisha told her brothers how she felt. The boys agreed to cut down on eating snacks at home. Mother and Keisha talked to the diabetes educator about adjusting Keisha's insulin and meal plan so that she could have occasional desserts and treats with her brothers.

YOUR TEEN WITH DIABETES

The teen years are often a challenging time for both youngsters and parents. As teenagers move toward adulthood they go through many physical and emotional changes. Their increasing maturity and desire for greater independence can affect their diabetes care and strain relationships with their parents.

Teens and Diabetes Care

For the teenager with diabetes, having to take insulin, test blood glucose regularly, and stick to a meal plan can all compound the normal difficulties of puberty. It's tempting for many teens to ease up on diabetes care and try to act like everyone else.

The teenage years are a period of developing a new identity. Many teens try to distance themselves from their families. Teens with diabetes may try to show their independence by

- refusing to do blood tests
- making up false test results
- bingeing on sweets or fatty foods like French fries and potato chips
- skipping insulin to lose weight

Parents are often shocked, baffled, and worried by this behavior. However, stay involved and interested in your teen's care. Your teen may be likely to take care of himself if he knows he is being supported and supervised.

If a teen and his parents are having a lot of problems related to diabetes care, an adult from outside the family (a coach, teacher, or nurse) may be able to provide the support the teen needs to manage his own care.

Setting realistic goals is important. If a teenager is only doing one blood test a day, negotiating with him to do two—and prais-

Sixteen-year-old Bob had a very busy schedule with school and sports and really couldn't do more than two blood tests a day. His mother scolded him for not doing more tests. At his most recent checkup he saw the diabetes educator, who said it was terrific that he did two blood tests a day. She didn't get upset or scold him. When she asked if Bob could try to do three tests on days when he played basketball, Bob thought he could handle that. With support and understanding, he had taken a step in the right direction.

ing him when he does it—will be more successful than demanding he do four.

Encouraging Independence

To help the teen with diabetes become independent, it is important to allow him to make decisions about his own care. Ideally, teens should already be making choices about meals and types and amounts of food. Remember, you're not going to be the one taking care of his diabetes when he's an adult—he is.

Let go gradually and allow the teen to take responsibility, as he feels ready, for blood testing and insulin injections. Your teen will make mistakes, but he will learn valuable lessons from them. You can help by making sure that proper supplies and foods are available.

Show that you are still interested and concerned about your teen by asking: "How are your tests running these days?" This shows that you expect your teen to be taking care of himself, but that you want to remain involved in his care.

Encourage your teen to develop a separate relationship with his doctor, dietitian, or diabetes educator. This can help him to find a treatment plan that he can live with. You can, of course, still talk to the doctor about concerns that you may have, but suggest that your teenager see his health care providers without you being present.

Try to be as loving, supportive, and patient as possible. It won't be easy, but many parents whose children don't have diabetes face similar problems. When the stresses of the teenage years seem to be creating great distress, psychological counseling may be helpful for teens and families. (See *Asking for Help*, page 140.) But most teens weather these stormy years quite well and become successful, self-assured adults.

Alcohol Use

Teenagers often want to try new and different things. Experimenting with alcohol is very common, even though it is illegal for teenagers to drink.

Alcohol poses special risks for people with diabetes. Drinking too much alcohol can lower blood glucose. Combining alcohol with a sugary mixer or with too much food can raise blood glucose.

Alcohol can cloud judgment. A teen who has been drinking may forget his care plan or neglect to treat low blood glucose. He may think that alcohol is making him feel strange when the feeling may be partly caused by plummeting blood glucose levels. Other people may not notice the signs of low blood glucose and think, "He's just drunk."

If a teen, knowing the risks to his diabetes control, decides to drink alcohol, he should be aware of the guidelines in the box on the next page.

Tobacco Use

Using tobacco in any form increases health risks. Smoking is linked to about 106,000 lung cancer deaths and about 225,000 heart disease deaths every year. Smoking can also cause high blood pressure, allergies, and ear and sinus infections.

People with diabetes already have a higher than average risk of getting heart disease, high blood pressure, and kidney disease. Combining smoking with diabetes further increases an individual's chances of having health problems.

Some teens chew tobacco or use snuff, thinking that these habits are less hazardous to health than smoking. In fact, the body absorbs more nicotine when tobacco is chewed or inhaled than when it is smoked. Chewing tobacco and snuff can make the nose and eyes run, cause irritation of the membranes in the nose and mouth, and lead to cancer of the nose and mouth.

In spite of these health risks, however, many teens choose to smoke or chew tobacco. Parents can help teens to decide against smoking by making the facts available—and by not smoking or chewing tobacco themselves.

When a person with diabetes tries to cut down on smoking or quit completely, he may experience symptoms of nicotine with-

GUIDELINES FOR ALCOHOL USE BY PEOPLE WITH DIABETES

Many adults with diabetes who drink moderately follow these guidelines.

- Know the harmful effects of alcohol. It's safest not to drink.
- Always carry your medical ID.
- If you can, make your own drink. That way, you'll know how much alcohol is in it.
- Have no more than two drinks.
- Make sure that at least one person with you knows that you have diabetes and knows the signs of low blood glucose.
- Check your blood glucose from time to time. This is particularly important if you are doing anything physically active like dancing, playing ball, or swimming.
- Drink slowly. Sometimes one drink can satisfy a craving and allow you to feel part of the crowd.
- The less alcohol in a drink, the better. Know the alcohol content of various kinds of liquor. Light wines often have low alcohol contents. Dry wines often have less sugar than sweeter ones.
- Alcohol has no nutritional benefits. For practical purposes, however, it is usually counted as a fat (1 oz alcohol = 1 Fat Exchange).
- Alcohol may make you hungry, and you may forget the importance of sticking to your meal plan. When drinking, try to avoid bingeing on party snacks and desserts.
- If you have a mixed drink, avoid sugar-sweetened mixers. Mix alcohol with water, diet soda, or club soda to dilute it.
- Alcohol is safest when consumed as a part of a meal or scheduled snack. Don't substitute alcohol for meals or snacks and don't drink on an empty stomach. If your meal is delayed, or you drink too much alcohol, you may have a low.
- Drinking and driving may be especially dangerous for people with diabetes. This is because alcohol may increase your risk of getting low blood glucose.
- If you are taking any medications such as antihistamines or cold remedies, talk to your doctor about what effect they may have on alcohol or on your diabetes control.

drawal (drowsiness, restless sleep, irritability, headache, and hunger) that are similar to symptoms of low blood glucose. Smoking cessation classes offered by high schools or community hospitals can be a source of support for those who are trying to give up tobacco use.

Illegal Drug Use

Some teens are attracted to illegal drugs like marijuana and cocaine. They may believe that these drugs are safe and that drug use is fun or a sign of maturity.

Before teens with diabetes consider using illegal drugs, they should know not only their general risks but also the special risks drugs pose to people with diabetes. Like alcohol, drugs can play havoc with blood glucose levels. In some case drugs lower glucose levels and in other cases raise them. A person's response to a drug may mask the warning signs of low blood glucose.

Marijuana can make people very hungry. Eating too much can, of course, cause high blood glucose levels and weight gain. Marijuana use can also lead to an attitude of indifference, which affects the way a teen manages diabetes, and diabetes control can deteriorate.

It may be hard for parents to get this information across effectively. One approach may be to provide booklets about drug use that are written especially for teenagers and that suggest resources teenagers can turn to for help or additional information.

Try to keep the lines of communication open. Find a quiet moment to have a calm discussion about drugs with your teen and listen to what he has to say. You might tell him that you understand his curiosity about drugs and the pressure he may be under to try them. However, research has shown that teens who do not use drugs have made this decision partly because of parental influence. Their common response is "my parents would *kill* me!" So it is very important to stand firmly against drug use, and equally important to stay very aware of your child's activities and involved in his life.

Driving

Getting a driver's license is a big day in every teen's life. Driving should not be a problem for the teen with diabetes, but he will need a doctor's clearance and should always be prepared for low blood glucose when driving.

Any driver with diabetes should always test his blood glucose before driving, unless he has just eaten. Your teen should always keep glucose gel or tablets, sugar cubes, and packaged crackers in the glove compartment of his car. You never know when a traffic jam could delay a meal or snack! If your teen feels a low blood glucose episode coming on while driving, he should park the car right away, treat the low, and wait until his blood glucose level returns to normal.

Driving may be a problem for a person with diabetes who does not feel early warning signs of low blood glucose. This is called *hypoglycemia unawareness*. Blood glucose testing before driving and at 2-hour intervals is essential for anyone who has this problem. Wearing an ID tag is important in case of an accident. (See *Should My Child Wear a Medical ID Tag?* page 84.)

Dating

Diabetes should not prevent a teen from having a full and fun-filled social life. For most teens, this will include dating. How to handle dating issues, however, is sometimes a concern. Teens have devised many successful approaches to handling diabetes while dating.

Your teen may wish to tell his date about diabetes. A brief explanation in advance may help him avoid alcohol or sweets at a party or clear the way for having a needed snack while out on a date. Explaining the signs of low blood glucose can help to prevent misunderstanding if your teen becomes irritable, pale, or restless.

Snacks should not be a problem on a date or at a party as long as they are included in his meal plan. Your teen can ask what food is being served at a party or discuss the choice of restaurant with his date beforehand. This allows time for him to adjust his meal plan. Some teens bring their own sugar-free soft drinks to parties or a platter of cut fresh vegetables to the snack table.

Eating Disorders

Eating disorders most often affect teenage girls and young women. A girl who is preoccupied with her weight or who feels she has no control over her life may be more likely to develop an eating disorder. Teenagers with diabetes may be at risk for eating disorders because they must focus on food and their meal plan. Because there are times when they must eat or drink, it may be harder for them to keep their weight under control.

The two most common eating disorders in teenage girls and young women are:

- **Anorexia nervosa.** People with this disorder lose weight by starving themselves.
- **Bulimia.** People with this disorder sometimes starve themselves and sometimes go on food binges. After bingeing, they may make themselves throw up or take laxatives or water pills to purge the food and water. A teenager with diabetes who binges and then skips her insulin, wreaks havoc on her blood glucose levels and metabolism in order to not gain weight.

A teenager who displays several of the following signs may have an eating disorder:

- extreme thinness
- wearing of multiple layers of clothing to cover what is perceived as fat
- cracks or redness in the corners of the mouth
- dark marks on the teeth, which indicate erosion of the tooth enamel

- a callous on the third knuckle, which may be caused by using the finger to induce vomiting
- trips to the bathroom after meals or snacks
- preoccupation with food or exercise
- weight loss or decreased insulin dose without an explanation
- depression

Eating disorders can be life-threatening. If you suspect that your teenager is developing an eating disorder or skipping insulin, notify your doctor right away.

Puberty and Sexual Development

Puberty produces many physical and hormonal changes as your child's body becomes that of an adult. Boys' bodies begin producing testosterone (the male sex hormone), which causes muscle development, growth of facial and body hair, and deepening of the voice. In girls, estrogen (the female sex hormone) causes menstruation and the growth of breasts and pubic hair.

These physical changes may be accompanied by emotional changes such as moodiness and irritability. Teens also usually begin to develop an interest in the opposite sex.

All children and teens grow and develop at different rates. Girls usually begin puberty at a younger age than boys do. Menstrual periods typically begin at age 12 to 13. However, heredity has a lot of influence on when your child reaches puberty. At 13 or 14, many boys are still boys while others are already becoming men.

Your son's growth and development will probably be similar to his father's and your daughter's will probably be similar to her mother's. For example, if Dad's voice changed at 15, Johnny's voice will probably change at around the same age. If Mom started having menstrual periods at 11, the chances are that Kerry will also start at that age.

If diabetes is well controlled it will not affect your child's growth and development. However, your doctor should carefully monitor your child's height, weight, and physical development.

Teens with diabetes, like other teenagers, may be sexually active. It's essential to talk to your teen honestly and directly about the risks of sex. Teach him about the likelihood of contracting sexually transmitted diseases such as the HIV virus, herpes, and syphilis; the risk of pregnancy; and available contraception. Send your teen the strong message that abstinence is the only certain way to avoid sexually transmitted diseases and pregnancy.

In many communities, you can get helpful information from the county health department or family planning clinics, where services are often both free and confidential. Your health care provider can help you find the county health department or family planning clinics in your area, if necessary.

Impotence (the inability to have an erection) can occur in men who have had diabetes for many years. It is extremely rare among teenage boys with diabetes, but fear of it may be present at an early age. Nerve damage caused by poor glucose control is one of the reasons men with diabetes become impotent. If your teenage son has concerns about this problem, a discussion with his doctor may help.

Career Choices

Many teenagers wonder, "Will diabetes limit my career choices?" The most honest answer to this question is "yes and no." By law, a person with type 1 diabetes cannot enlist in the military or pilot a commercial aircraft. With these exceptions, however, most occupations are open to people with diabetes.

Some laws excluding people with diabetes from certain types of work have been successfully challenged. For example, at one time people with diabetes could not drive commercial vehicles such as trucks or buses. Now, however, people with diabetes may be accepted as truck or bus drivers on a case-by-case basis.

People with diabetes are protected against job discrimination by many state and federal laws. A person who feels that he has been discriminated against may contact the American Diabetes

Association for further information about these laws and possible recourse against discrimination.

Advances in the treatment of diabetes have opened professional doors. People with diabetes are working in many careers, including police work and fire fighting. Like all people, teens with diabetes should choose careers based on their talents, interests, and qualifications.

People with diabetes are among the leading doctors, scientists, political leaders, teachers, and lawyers in the U.S. Celebrities and sports figures with diabetes include:

■ 1999 Miss America Nicole Johnson
■ actors Mary Tyler Moore, Jean Smart, and Wilfred Brimley
■ professional football players Jonathan Hayes and Wade Wilson
■ professional basketball player Chris Dudley
■ rock musician Bret Michaels

Marriage

Teenagers with diabetes may have concerns about marriage. Many people with diabetes are very happily married. However, the issues related to diabetes should be discussed with the prospective partner before the wedding takes place.

The partner of a person with diabetes may face some lifestyle changes. He or she must understand the need to take insulin, to stick to a meal plan, and to check blood glucose levels frequently. The partner may have to deal with mood swings that can occur with changes in blood glucose levels. Some partners may feel anxious about treating low blood glucose episodes. In many cases, partners can benefit from attending diabetes education classes.

Pregnancy

Diabetes need not prevent most women from having a family. Pregnancy does pose extra risks to both the woman with diabetes and her baby, but with good medical care women with diabetes give birth to healthy infants all the time.

Achieving good diabetes control *before* becoming pregnant is extremely important. Uncontrolled diabetes during the first few weeks of pregnancy can cause birth defects. Prenatal care and tight control of blood glucose levels during pregnancy help to assure the birth of a healthy baby.

Teenagers may wonder whether their children will also get diabetes. Research shows that some people do inherit a higher risk of getting diabetes. Recent studies show that of 100 children born to a parent with type 1 diabetes, between 1 and 8 may get diabetes. A couple in which one partner has diabetes may wish to get genetic counseling before starting a family.

Living with Diabetes

BUDGETING

Caring for a child with diabetes on a limited budget is a challenge, but it can be done. Your dietitian can give you some useful hints about how to prepare inexpensive, healthful meals for your entire family. As with food, when shopping for diabetes supplies, it helps to compare prices, use coupons, and buy in bulk.

Always compare prices of supplies before buying. Companies that offer mail order diabetes supplies will vary in price, selection, and service. It pays to shop around. Check the American Diabetes Association's magazine *Diabetes Forecast* for ads by companies that offer diabetes supplies in bulk by mail. The *Diabetes Forecast Resource Guide*, published every January, is a very useful source of information about different types of diabetes supplies and where to find them.

TRAVELING

Vacations and trips are special times. A trip means a break from school, work, and the everyday routine. Unfortunately, it doesn't mean a break from diabetes care. Diabetes never takes a vacation. The box on the next page provides useful tips that will help you to plan a safe and enjoyable vacation with a child with diabetes.

TIPS FOR TRAVELING—PART I

Before you go

■ If your child is taking a long trip, it's a good idea for her to have a complete medical checkup before leaving. Take a record of the checkup along on the trip. Important information in the record should include insulin dose and blood test results.

■ When making flight reservations, check the times that meals and snacks will be served. Airlines have special meals for people with diabetes. Ask for these when you make your reservations. It's a good idea to bring extra food like crackers or fruit in case the meals are delayed or do not appear.

■ If you are traveling to a different time zone, get advice from your health care provider about how to adjust the timing of meals, insulin injections, and so on.

Packing

■ Pack diabetes supplies so they are always within easy reach. When traveling by plane, take syringes and insulin in a carry-on bag. This protects you in case your luggage is lost.

■ Insulin need not be packed in a thermos or ice chest. But insulin bottles should be kept in a cool, dry place and protected from breakage. Insulin should not be exposed to extreme heat or cold, so don't pack it in the trunk of a hot car or keep it in the glove compartment.

■ Always carry an emergency kit for hypoglycemia (low blood glucose) with you when traveling. In the emergency kit should be:
  ● a fast-acting sugar (such as fruit juice, sugar cubes, or glucose tablets)
  ● a long-acting carbohydrate and protein (such as peanut butter or cheese crackers)
  ● a glucagon kit

■ Pack extra food, syringes, and insulin in a second bag in case one becomes lost.

■ Your child should wear a medical ID tag and you should carry a medical information packet (see *Should My Child Wear a Medical ID Tag?* on page 84). In your packet should be your physician's name and phone number, and spare prescriptions for insulin, syringes, and glucagon.

■ If you're traveling to a country where trafficking in illegal drugs is a concern, you may want to carry a letter from your child's doctor explaining her need for insulin and syringes.

SOLVING THE DAY TO DAY CHALLENGES OF DIABETES

Many times parents ask for advice on specific childhood challenges that crop up with diabetes. Two main areas of difficulty seem to exist for parents: helping their children deal with their feelings about having diabetes, and getting their kids to cooperate with diabetes care routines.

Dealing with Feelings

Many people will try to reassure you when you find out your child has diabetes. They will tell you that you can cope with this and that your child has every chance of living a full, normal life with diabetes. This may be true. But having diabetes is not normal, and doing diabetes care things like testing blood and giving shots is not an inherently pleasant part of a child's day. Having diabetes is not easy, and having angry or sad feelings about it is to be expected.

Dealing with your child's feelings can be difficult and painful. But having your child talk about feelings is important, especially with you. There are certain skills parents can use to encourage conversations about feelings with their children. To keep the communication going:

- listen with your full attention
- accept your child's feelings without denying them
- acknowledge with one word

Listen with your full attention. Many parents with busy schedules (especially when diabetes care is added in) do not find it easy to stop what they are doing to listen to their children. It

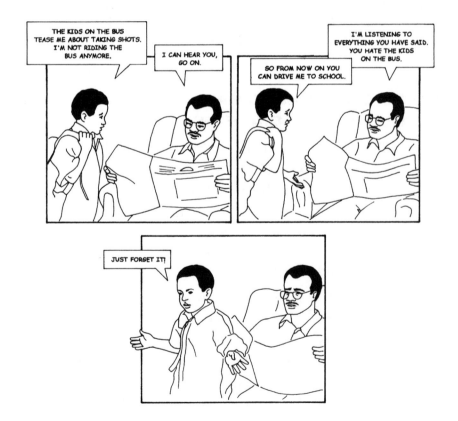

is discouraging for a child to try to get through to someone who is only half-listening. It is much more rewarding to tell your troubles to a parent who is really listening.

Careful listening is hard work. Many times parents are waiting for their children to finish talking so they can say what they want to say. Although it does require effort at the time, in the long run the time spent listening to your child will pay off. If your child comes to you with a concern, stop what you are doing, sit down, and listen. Sometimes, a parent doesn't need to say anything. Often an understanding silence is all the child needs to solve her own problems.

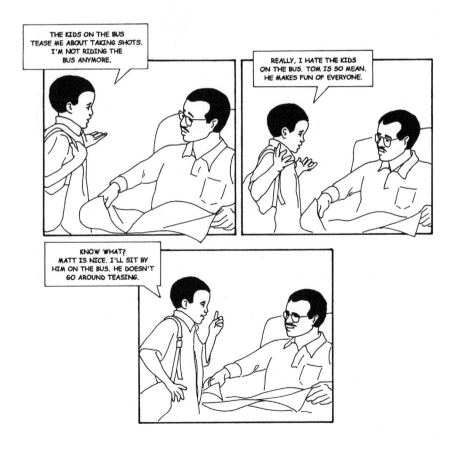

Accept your child's feelings without denying them. Try not to deny what your child is feeling. Sometimes parents feel so badly about the diabetes, they try to help their children by making diabetes seem like a smaller problem than it really is. In other words, parents are denying the way the child really feels. For example, saying things like, "You can handle it, there's no need to be upset," "It doesn't hurt that much!" and "It's not so bad" tell your child her feelings are not valid.

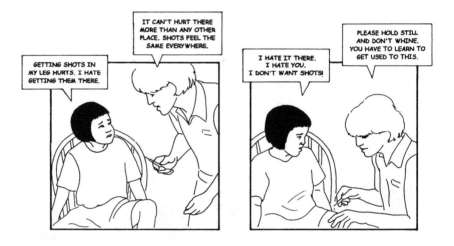

It's often easier for parents to understand how denying feelings affects communication when they put themselves in their child's place. For example, imagine if you were told to lose weight and needed to cut out desserts. You really enjoy desserts, and you share your frustration with a friend. Your friend responds by saying, "That's no big deal!" and "It's easy to avoid sweets." How would you feel?

You might feel angry or that your friend doesn't understand. You may think there is no point in talking to this friend again about your frustration. Wouldn't it have been easier to talk to your friend if she accepted your feelings? What if she had said, "It must be tough for you. I like desserts too. I would hate missing them."

Try to tune in to your child's true feelings, and helpful words will often come to you. For example, you may find yourself saying, "Wow! You must still be hungry, even though you just had lunch," or "I can see that this shot hurt a little more than usual," or "Eating carrots for a snack is fine for me, but I bet you would prefer something else."

Remember that you and your child are separate people, and probably feel very differently about things. Acknowledge your child's separate reality.

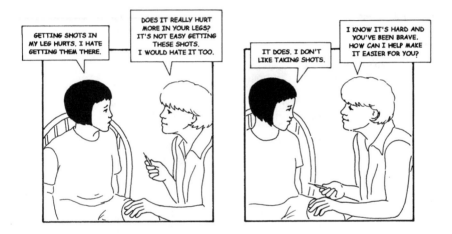

Acknowledge with one word. Instead of asking a lot of questions and giving advice, sometimes it is better to acknowledge your child's feelings with just a word. Children, especially teens, don't always appreciate questions or advice. It is hard for a child to think clearly about a problem if someone is blaming, criticizing, or giving advice. Phrases like "You know what I think you should do?" or "If you're smart you'll always carry glucose tablets with you, so nothing like this happens again," or "I keep telling you to keep your meter in the nurse's office. You lost it before!" are not helpful.

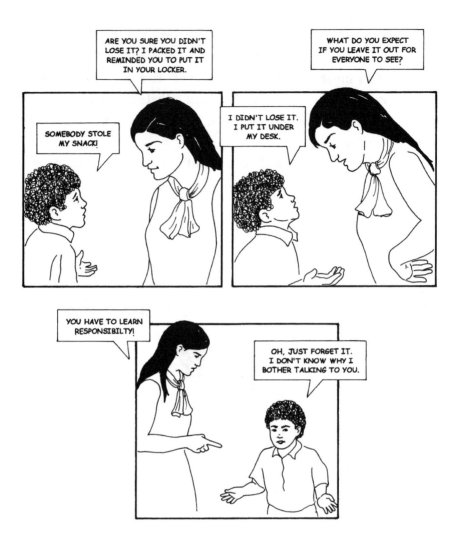

To get your child to continue talking about her feelings, sometimes it is helpful for a parent to simply say "Oh" or "Hmmm" or "I see." Words like these often open the door for your child to continue exploring his own thoughts.

There's a lot to be gained when parents allow their children to solve their own problems by encouraging them with simple words like "Oh?" or "Really." Words like these combined with a caring, listening approach are invitations for children to explore their own thoughts and find their own solutions.

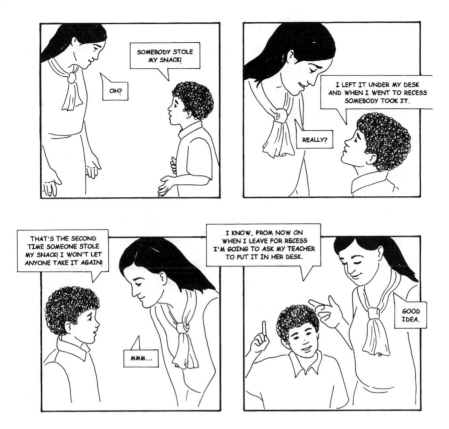

Getting Cooperation

One of the toughest jobs in being a parent is trying to get children to do what they are supposed to do. The daily struggles of getting children to make their beds, brush their teeth, do homework, or walk the dog are quite enough. With diabetes there are even more struggles: doing the blood tests, carrying snacks, giving shots, and so on.

Parents often complain that they feel like nags. Children often say their parents are slave drivers who have an endless stream of tedious tasks for them to do.

In getting children to cooperate, parents should think about the ways they have used to get their children to do their jobs.

Some parents blame or accuse: "How many times do I have to tell you to wash your hands before testing?" "You never wear your ID bracelet. I paid good money for that!" "The trouble with you is you never tell the doctor the truth!"

Some parents give commands: "I want you to record your blood sugars right now!" "Hurry up and take your shot—the bus is coming!" Some use warnings: "You better be careful or you'll end up in the hospital." "You better not do that again or you will go low." And other parents are martyrs: "I'm drained from dealing with all of this and you don't make it any easier." "Are you trying to give me a heart attack?"

There are alternatives to these common approaches that will ease the tension and will most likely result in more cooperation from your child. To get your child to cooperate with diabetes care routines:

- describe what you see, or describe the problem
- give information
- use fewer words
- talk about your feelings
- write a note

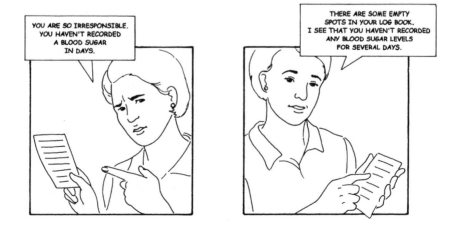

Describe what you see, or describe the problem. It's hard to think about what needs to be done when someone is telling you what's wrong with you. It's easier to think about the problem when someone describes it to you.

Give information. Information is a lot easier to take than accusation. When you give information, you are giving your child a gift. Isn't it better for your child to know there is a way to eat candy openly instead of hiding it and feeling ashamed or guilty?

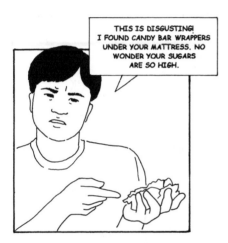
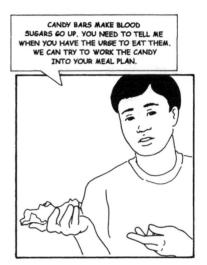

Use fewer words. In this case, less is more.

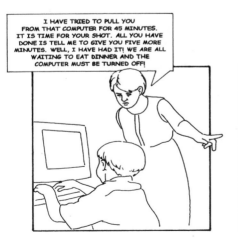
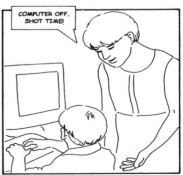

Talk about your feelings. Instead of commenting on your child's character or personality, talk about how you feel.

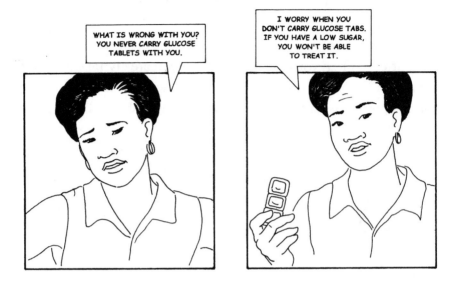

Write a note. Sometimes there is nothing more effective than writing down what you want in a note.

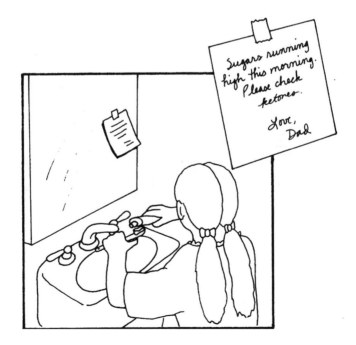

COPING WITH DIABETES

Having a child with diabetes can at times be very stressful for you and your family. It can be hard at first to accept that your child has a disease that isn't going to go away and that needs care and attention every day. Caring for a child with diabetes alters your family routine and can affect relationships among family members.

Having diabetes is stressful for your child, too. Young children may think that diabetes is a punishment for something they did. It's important to try to reassure your child that having diabetes isn't her fault.

Feeling loved by the whole family can help your child to accept having diabetes. Involving everyone in the family in your child's care can help to make diabetes a normal part of family life.

Parents often worry about disciplining a child with diabetes because it can be hard to tell the difference between normal misbehavior and signs of low blood glucose. It's important, however, not to treat your child with diabetes differently from your other children. Ordinary discipline should not have any effect on your child's blood glucose levels.

ASKING FOR HELP

Every family will go through times when it's hard to cope with the demands of diabetes on top of the stresses of everyday life. During these difficult periods, you and your family may benefit from the help of a professional counselor.

Professional counselors are trained to help people with special problems and concerns. Many people are ashamed to ask for this kind of help. Some think that asking for help makes them a failure. Others fear being labeled mentally ill.

These concerns are understandable, but unjustified. There is no shame in asking for help to cope with a very hard job that gives you no time off. Caring for a child with diabetes is exactly such a job. Knowing when you need extra help is a sign of mental health, not mental illness.

Counseling can make a real difference in how diabetes affects you and your child. Many families find that just one session with a counselor makes a big difference.

How do you find a counselor that you like and feel comfortable with? If a health care team cares for your child, the team may include a counselor (a social worker, psychologist, or psychiatrist). Your child's doctor may be able to refer you to a good counselor. Many communities have family service organizations that offer counseling.

You may want to go to a meeting of a support group affiliated with the American Diabetes Association. These groups usually meet informally. They offer a chance for your child to meet other children with diabetes and for you to meet other parents of children with diabetes. Parents can exchange experiences, problems, and solutions. Families can see that they are not alone. Other families are facing similar challenges—and surviving.

Look in your telephone book to see if there is an American Diabetes Association chapter in your area. The American Diabetes Association also has many books, pamphlets, and other publications about diabetes available (see *Resources*, page 155).

CONCLUSION

Living successfully with diabetes isn't always easy, but with discipline, patience, and good medical care, it can be done. Everything about life with diabetes is a balancing act. You have to balance food, insulin, and activity to keep blood glucose levels within a target range.

Your child with diabetes depends on you for care and support. He will follow your lead. If you can feel comfortable and positive about your child's condition, he will learn to feel the same way. If you have a can-do attitude when faced with life's surprises, he'll take on challenges with the same outlook.

When your child is very young, you will do all of the day-to-day tasks of caring for his diabetes. As your child grows up, it's important that he gradually learns to take on these tasks for himself. But it's also important that you stay involved in your child's care even as you let your child take on more responsibility. This, too, is a balancing act.

The child who learns to live with diabetes has to do many things that other children don't have to do and make many decisions that other children don't have to make. He learns early in life the importance of being disciplined and taking responsibility for himself.

These are lessons that can prepare your child for life as an adult. No one would choose to have diabetes in order to learn these things. But learning to live successfully with diabetes can, ultimately, be an experience that enriches your child's whole life.

Glossary

Adrenaline: A hormone that helps the body deal with stress. By making the body produce more glucose, adrenaline can raise the blood glucose level.

Antibody: A protein made in response to a bacteria or virus that fights infection.

Autoimmune disorder: A disease in which antibodies, instead of helping the body fight infection, attack normal parts of the body. For example, antibodies may attack and destroy the cells that make insulin, causing diabetes.

Beta cells: Small clumps of cells in the pancreas that make insulin. In type 1 diabetes, these cells are destroyed and no longer can produce insulin.

Carbohydrate: The body's preferred source of energy. There are two kinds of carbohydrates: **simple sugars,** which the body processes quickly, and **complex carbohydrates,** which generally take more time to digest. Simple sugars cause a rapid rise in the blood glucose level. Complex carbohydrates tend to cause a more gradual rise in blood glucose.

Cardiovascular: Relating to the heart and blood vessels.

Cell: The basic structural unit of all animals and plants. Cells are the physical basis of all life processes.

Cell membrane: Material that surrounds each cell. The membrane keeps in substances that the cell needs and excludes harmful ones.

Diabetes educator: A health care professional who has specialized training in the care of diabetes. A diabetes educator may be a nurse, a dietitian, a pharmacist, a social worker, a physician, or may be trained in another health care field. A **Certified Diabetes Educator (CDE)** has passed a qualifying exam and has spent a specific amount of time teaching people about diabetes.

Diabetic coma: See **ketoacidosis**.

Dietitian: A health care professional who has specialized training in diet and nutrition. A Registered Dietitian (RD) has passed a qualifying exam.

Endocrinologist: A physician who specializes in the treatment of diseases caused by imbalances of hormones. Diabetes is one such disease. Some endocrinologists who specialize in treating patients with diabetes call themselves **diabetologists**.

Exchange Lists: A meal planning tool for people with diabetes. Exchange Lists divide food into six categories: starch, meat, vegetable, fruit, milk, and fat. Each list consists of foods that, in the stated amounts, can be "exchanged" or substituted for any other food on the same list.

Fats: A food group and a source of energy for the body. Fats do not raise blood glucose very much, but some kinds of fat raise the cholesterol level in the blood.

> **Saturated fat:** Fat that tends to raise the cholesterol level in the blood. Usually found in foods that come from animals. Butter and lard are saturated fats. Some vegetable oils, such as palm oil and coconut oil, are also saturated fats.

> **Monounsaturated fat:** Fat that tends to lower blood cholesterol. Olive oil and canola oil are monounsaturated fats.

Polyunsaturated fat: Fat that tends to lower blood cholesterol. Found in most vegetable oils. Soybean oil, cottonseed oil, corn oil, and peanut oil are all polyunsaturated fats.

Gingivitis: Inflammation of the gums. Gingivitis can be a long-term complication of diabetes, but it can be reduced or prevented with regular dental care.

Glucagon: A hormone produced in the pancreas. Glucagon raises blood glucose levels. It is also given by injection for treating very low blood glucose if a person cannot eat or drink.

Glucose: A kind of sugar. Glucose is the body's main source of energy. The digestive system makes glucose by breaking down carbohydrate.

Glycated hemoglobin: A substance in red blood cells. Also called HbA. The HbA_{1c} test shows what the average blood glucose level has been over the past couple of months.

Glycemic response: The rate and amount by which a certain food raises blood glucose.

Glycosuria: Glucose in the urine.

Hormone: A substance made by an endocrine gland that aids growth or body functioning. Adrenaline, glucagon, and insulin are hormones.

Hyperglycemia: A high level of glucose in the blood. Common symptoms include frequent urination, excessive thirst, weight loss, increased appetite, tiredness, and blurred vision. Hyperglycemia is a sign of uncontrolled diabetes. It may be treated by giving a bigger dose of insulin or by getting exercise to lower blood glucose levels. Untreated, hyperglycemia can lead to **ketoacidosis**.

Hyperlipidemia: A high level of fats in the blood.

Hypoglycemia: A low level of glucose in the blood. Common symptoms include nervousness, headache, pallor, fatigue, weakness, nightmares, hunger, irritability, sweating, personality changes, shakiness, and confusion. Hypoglycemia must be treated quickly.

Untreated, it can lead to seizures and unconsciousness. Treat hypoglycemia with sugar to raise blood glucose levels quickly.

Insulin: A hormone made in the beta cells of the pancreas. It allows the body to use glucose for energy.

Insulin resistance: A condition common in type 2 diabetes, where the body is unable to use circulating insulin.

Islets of Langerhans: Clusters of cells in the pancreas. The islets are made of four kinds of cells. **Beta cells** are the ones that make insulin.

Juvenile-onset diabetes: Former name for insulin-dependent diabetes or type 1 diabetes. This term is no longer used.

Ketoacidosis: A serious condition that means diabetes is uncontrolled. Ketones, byproducts of fat digestion, build up in the body, creating acidity in the blood. Symptoms include nausea, vomiting, fruity-smelling breath, dry skin, labored breathing, and stupor, which can lead to **diabetic coma.** Usually occurs at diagnosis, or with flu or illness.

Ketone: A waste product made by the body when it burns fat for energy.

Ketonemia: Ketones in the blood.

Ketonuria: Ketones in the urine.

Kidney: One of a pair of organs that functions to remove waste products from the blood by filtering them into the urine.

Lipids: Complex fats used in the body to store and transport needed minerals.

Lispro (Humalog): A rapid-acting insulin that can be injected just before meals.

Maturity-onset diabetes: Former name for type 2 diabetes. This term is no longer used.

Metabolic rate: The rate at which the body performs its chemical and physical functions.

Metabolism: All of the chemical and physical changes in the body that enable it to grow and function.

Minerals: Substances needed in small amounts to build and repair body tissues and/or to control functions of the body. Calcium, iron, potassium, and magnesium are examples of minerals.

Nephropathy: Kidney disease. People who have had diabetes for many years are at risk of getting nephropathy.

Neuropathy: Nerve disease. Often causes loss of sensation or movement and pain or burning in the feet and legs. May also affect nerves in other parts of the body. People who have had diabetes for many years and/or poor blood glucose control are at risk of getting neuropathy.

Nutrient: A substance in food that is needed by the body. Proteins, fats, carbohydrates, minerals, vitamins, and water are examples of nutrients.

Ophthalmologist: A medical doctor who specializes in the care and treatment of eye diseases.

Optometrist: A specialist who is trained to examine the eyes and prescribe lenses or exercises to correct vision problems.

Pancreas: An organ that produces insulin, digestive enzymes, and other hormones.

Polydipsia: Increased thirst. A symptom of **hyperglycemia**.

Polyphagia: Increased appetite. A symptom of **hyperglycemia**. Can also accompany hypoglycemia.

Polyuria: Increased urination. A symptom of **hyperglycemia**.

Protein: A nutrient found in food. Proteins are building blocks and a source of energy.

Psychologist: A health care professional who has specialized training in the treatment of problems that cause mental and emotional distress.

Retinopathy: A disease of the retina in the eye. A complication of diabetes.

Signs: An abnormal finding, such as fever based on a thermometer reading.

Social worker: A person with specialized training in helping individuals and families to solve practical and emotional problems.

Symptoms: An abnormal sensation or physical complaint, such as abdominal pain.

Type 1 diabetes: An autoimmune disease where the pancreas makes insufficient insulin.

Type 2 diabetes: A disease where the body is unable to use insulin properly.

Vitamins: Substances needed in small amounts for normal body growth and functioning.

Resources

Some of the resources listed below are for all people with diabetes, not just children. They are included here because you may have another family member with diabetes, or you may find them helpful later.

Some of the ADA books listed after the Index are particularly helpful for children with diabetes. Look for:

- *The Dinosaur Tamer*
- *The Take-Charge Guide to Type 1 Diabetes*
- *The Ten Keys to Helping Your Child Grow Up with Diabetes*
- *Sweet Kids: How to Balance Diabetes Control & Good Nutrition with Family Peace*

You might also find the following titles helpful:

- *Psyching Out Diabetes* by Richard Rubin, June Biermann, and Barbara Toohey (Lowell House)
- *Don't Shoot the Dog* by Karen Pryor (Bantam Books)
- *Time to Learn About Diabetes* by Jean Betschart (Wiley & Sons)
- *A Magic Ride in Foozbah Land: An Inside Look at Diabetes* by Jean Betschart (Wiley & Sons)
- *In Control: A Guide for Teens* by Jean Betschart (Wiley & Sons)
- *Diabetes Care for Babies, Toddlers, and Preschoolers: A Reassuring Guide* by Jean Betschart and Sue Thom (Wiley & Sons)

FOR FINDING QUALITY HEALTH CARE

American Association for Marriage and Family Therapy
1133 15th Street NW, Suite 300
Washington, DC 20005-2710

For marriage and family therapists in your area, send a self-addressed, stamped envelope to the attention of Mr. Johnson.

American Association of Diabetes Educators
444 North Michigan Avenue
Suite 1240
Chicago, IL 60611
312–644–2233
312–644–4411 (fax)
800–832–6874

Referral to a local diabetes educator.

American Association of Sex Educators, Counselors, and Therapists
P.O. Box 238
Mount Vernon, IA 52314-0238

For a list of certified sex therapists and counselors in your state, send a self-addressed, stamped, business-size envelope (you may request lists from more than one state).

American Board of Medical Specialties
47 Perimeter Center East
Suite 500
Atlanta, GA 30346
800–776–2378

Record of physicians certified by 24 medical specialty boards. Only certification status of physician is available to callers. Directories of certified physicians organized by city of medical practice and alphabetically by physician names are available in many libraries.

American Board of Podiatric Surgery
1601 Dolores Street
San Francisco, CA 94110
415–826–3200
415–826–4640 (fax)

Referral to a local board-certified podiatrist.

The American Dietetic Association
216 West Jackson Boulevard
Suite 800
Chicago, IL 60606
312–899–0040
312–899–1979 (fax)
800–366–1655 Consumer Nutrition Hot Line; 9–4 CST, M–F only

Information, guidance, and referral to a local dietitian.

American Medical Association
515 North State Street
Chicago, IL 60610
312–464–4818
Web site: http://www.ama–assn.org

Referral to your county or state medical society, which may be able to refer you to a local physician.

American Optometric Association
243 N. Lindbergh Boulevard
St. Louis, MO 63141
314–991–4100
314–991–4101 (fax)
Web site: http://www.aoanet.org \ aoanet

Referral to your state optometric association for referral to a local optometrist.

American Psychiatric Association
1400 K Street NW
Washington, DC 20005
202–682–6000
202–682–6114 (fax)
Web site: http://www.psych.org

Referral to your state psychiatric association for referral to a local psychiatrist.

American Psychological Association
750 First Street NE
Washington, DC 20002-4242
202-336-5500 (main number)
202-336-5700 (public affairs)
202-436-5800 (professional practice)
Web site: http://www.apa.org

Referral to your state psychological
association for referral to a local
psychologist.

National Association of Social Workers
750 First Street NE, Suite 700
Washington, DC 20002-4247
202-408-8600
800-638-8799

Referral to your state chapter of NASW
for referral to a local social worker.

Pedorthic Footwear Association
9861 Broken Land Parkway, Suite 255
Columbia, MD 21046-1151
410-381-7278
410-381-1167 (fax)
800-673-8447

Referral to a local certified pedorthist (a
person trained in fitting prescription
footwear).

FOR MISCELLANEOUS HEALTH INFORMATION

American Academy of Ophthalmology
Customer Service Department
655 Beach Street
San Francisco, CA 94109-1336
415-561-8500
415-561-8533 (fax)
Web site: http://www.eyenet.org

For brochures on eye care and eye
diseases, send a self-addressed, stamped
envelope.

American Heart Association
7272 Greenville Avenue
Dallas, TX 75231
800-242-8721
Web site: http://www.amhrt.org

For referral to local affiliate's *Heartline*,
which provides information on
cardiovascular health and disease
prevention.

Impotence World Association
10400 Little Patuxent Parkway
Suite 485
Columbia, MD 21044
410-715-9609
800-669-1603

For information and guidance on
impotence and physician referral in your
state, send a written request and $2.00
for postage and handling.

Medic Alert Foundation
P.O. Box 1009
Turlock, CA 95381-1009
209-668-3331
209-669-2495 (fax)
800-432-5378
Web site: http://www.medicalert.org

To order a medical ID bracelet.

National AIDS Hot Line
Centers for Disease Control and
    Prevention
800-342-2437 (24 hours)
800-344-7432 (Spanish)
800-243-7889 (TTY)

Information on HIV and AIDS,
including pamphlets and brochures,
counseling, and referral to local test sites,
case managers, and medical services.

National Chronic Pain Outreach Association
P.O. Box 274
Millboro, VA 24460
540–997–5004
540–997–1305 (fax)
e-mail: ncpoal@aol.com
To learn more about chronic pain and how to deal with it.

National Kidney Foundation
30 E. 33rd Street
New York, NY 10016
212–889–2210
212–689–9261 (fax)
800–622–9010
Web site: http://www.mcw.edu/nkf

For donor cards and information about kidney disease and transplants.

United Network for Organ Sharing
1100 Boulders Parkway, Suite 500
P.O. Box 13770
Richmond, VA 23225-8770
804-330-8602 (communications)
800–355–SHARE (for information on becoming a donor)
800–24–DONOR

For information about organ transplants and a list of organ transplant centers in the U.S.

FOR TRAVELERS

U.S. Government Printing Office
Superintendent of Documents
P.O. Box 371954
Pittsburgh, PA 15250-7954
202–512–1800
202–512–2250 (fax)

Order the brochure *Health Information for International Travelers* (stock # 017–023–001957) by phone with credit card or send check or money order for $14.

International Association for Medical Assistance to Travelers
417 Center Street
Lewiston, NY 14092
716–754–4883
519–836–3412 (fax)

For a list of doctors in foreign countries who speak English and who received postgraduate training in North America or Great Britain.

International Diabetes Federation
40 Washington Street
B–1050 Brussels, Belgium

For a list of International Diabetes Federation groups that can offer assistance when you're traveling.

FOR EXERCISERS

American College of Sports Medicine
P.O. Box 1440
Indianapolis, IN 46206-1440
317–637–9200
317–634–7817 (fax)
Web site: http://www.acsm.org/sportsmed

For information about health and fitness.

International Diabetic Athletes Association
1647 W. Bethany Home Road, #B
Phoenix, AZ 85015-2507
800–898–IDAA
e-mail: idaa@getnet.com
Web site: http://www.getnet.com/~idaa/

For people with diabetes and for health care professionals interested in exercise and fitness at all levels. Newsletter.

President's Council on Physical Fitness and Sports
701 Pennsylvania Avenue NW
Suite 250
Washington, DC 20004
202–272–3421
202–504–2064 (fax)

For information about physical activity, exercise, and fitness.

FOR EQUAL EMPLOYMENT INFORMATION

American Bar Association
Commission on Mental and Physical
    Disability Law
740 15th Street NW
Washington, DC 20005-1009
202–662–1570
202–662–1032 (fax)
202–662–1012 (TTY)
Web site: http://www.abanet.org/disability

Provides information and technical assistance on all aspects of disability law.

Disability Rights Education and Defense Fund, Inc.
2212 6th Street
Berkeley, CA 94710
510–644–2555 (voice/TDD)
510–841–8645 (fax)
800–466–4232 (voice/TDD)
e-mail: dredfca@aol.com

Provides technical assistance and information to employers and individuals with disabilities on disability rights legislation and policies. Assists with legal representation.

Equal Employment Opportunity Commission
1801 L Street NW
Washington, DC 20507
For technical assistance and filing a
    charge:
202–663–4900
202–663–4912 (fax)
800–669–4000 (connects to nearest local
    EEOC office)
800–669–3362 (for publications)
800–800–3302 (TDD)

National Information Center for Children and Youth With Disabilities
P.O. Box 1492
Washington, DC 20013-1492
202–884–8200 (voice and TDD)
202–884–8441 (fax)
800–695–0285 (voice and TTY)
Web site: http://www.aed.org/nichcy

Provides technical assistance and information on disabilities and disability-related issues.

FOR HEALTH INSURANCE INFORMATION

AARP health insurance
800–523–5800

The AARP administers 10 health insurance plans. For some plans, individuals with diabetes or other chronic illnesses are eligible within 6 months after enrolling in Medicare Part B. For other plans, a 3-month waiting period is required for those with conditions preexistent in the 6 months preceding the effective date of the insurance, if not replacing previous coverage.

Medicare Hot Line
800–638–6833
U.S. Department of Health and Human
Services
Health Care Financing Administration
6325 Security Boulevard
Baltimore, MD 21207

For information and various publications
about Medicare.

Social Security Administration
800–772–1213

For information and various publications
about Medicare.

HELPFUL WEB SITES

www.diabetes.org (ADA Web site)

www.diabeteswebsite.com (site of
popular authors and diabetes men-
tors June Biermann and Barbara
Toohey)

www.niddk.nih.gov/health/
diabetes/diabetes.htm (NIH/
NIDDK government Web site)

www.childrenwithdiabetes.
com (created by a father; offers many
chat rooms and answers to more
than 3,000 questions on-line)

www.diabetesmonitor.com (supplies
information on upcoming medications and research, plus a mentor
section)

www.mendosa.com/diabetes.
htm (a diabetes dictionary)

dnet.ori.org/newuser (Oregon
Research Institute's diabetes network)

www.diabetes.com
(lots of news from medical journals)
www.diabetes.fyi.net (order books
and a video by Jean Betschart)

You can also subscribe to the following list servers (groups of people who
share information about a topic):

listserv@lehigh.edu. To subscribe,
send an e-mail to the list serve. In
the message box write the words
"subscribe diabetic your name"
(write your name here).

majordomo@world.std.com. To subscribe, send an e-mail to the list
serve. In the message box write the
words "subscribe diabetes".

ADA REGIONAL OFFICES

New England Region
7 Washington Square
Albany, NY 12205
518/218-1755
Joyce Waite, Regional
    Executive Vice President

Massachusetts Area Office
617/482-4580

Northern New England Area Office
603/627-9579

Rhode Island Area Office
401/738-6464

Pacific Northwest Region
2480 West 26th Avenue
Suite 120B
Denver, CO 80211
720/855-1102
Mike Van Abel, Regional Executive
    Vice President

Alaska Area Office
907/272-1424

Hawaii Area Office
808/521-1142

Idaho Area Office
208/342-2774

Montana Area Office
406/761-0908

Oregon Area Office
503/736-2770

Washington Area Office
206/352-7950

South Central Region
4425 West Airport Freeway
Suite 130
Irving, TX 75062
972/255-6900
Quincy Neal, Regional
    Executive Vice President

Arkansas Area Office
501/221-7444

Louisiana Area Office
504/831-0278

Northeast Texas/Northern Louisiana
Area Office
972/392-1181

Oklahoma Area Office
918/492-3839

South Texas Area Office
210/829-1765

West Texas Area Office
806/794-0691

South Coastal Region
1101 North Lake Destiny Road
Suite 415
Maitland, FL 32751
407/660-1926
Nancy Carlton, Regional Executive
    Vice President

Atlanta Metro Area Office
404/320-7100

Central Florida Area Office
407/660-1926

Northeast Florida/Southeast Georgia
Area Office
904/703-7200

Northwest Florida/Southern
Alabama Area Office
850/478-5957

Outstate Georgia Area Office
912/353-8110

Southeast Florida Area Office
305/477-8999

Southwest Florida Area Office
813/885-5007

Upstate Alabama Area Office
205/870-5172

Southern Region
2 Hanover Square
434 Fayetteville Square Mall
Suite 1600
Raleigh, NC 27601
919/743-5400
Edward L. Owens, Regional
    Executive Vice President

Central North Carolina Area Office
704/373-9111

Eastern North Carolina Area Office
919/743-5400

Greater Hampton Roads Area Office
757/455-6335

Kentucky Area Office
502/452-6072

South Carolina Area Office
803/799-4246

Tennessee Area Office
615/298-3066

Virginia Area Office
804/974-9905

Western Region
10445 Old Placerville Road
Sacramento, CA 95827-2508
916/369-0999
Michael Clinkenbeard, Regional
    Executive Vice President

Los Angeles Area Office
213/966-2890

Nevada Area Office
702/369-9995

Sacramento Area Office
916/369-0999

San Diego Area Office
619/234-9897

San Francisco Area Office
510/654-4499

Index

Books from the American Diabetes Association

Self-Care

New!

The American Diabetes Association
Complete Guide to Diabetes, 2nd Edition
American Diabetes Association

Everything you ever needed to know about diabetes contained inside one practical book—now updated! One of the most complete and authoritative resources you can find on diabetes, it covers everything from how to manage types 1 and 2 and gestational diabetes to traveling with insulin, sick day action plans, and recognizing hypoglycemia. You get in-depth coverage on preventing and treating complications, recognizing symptoms, exercising, nutrition, glucose control, sexual issues, pregnancy, and more.

One Low Price: $23.95
Order #4809-02

New!

The Diabetes Problem Solver

Nancy Touchette, PhD

Quick: You think you may have diabetic ketoacidosis, a life-threatening condition. What are the symptoms? What should you do first? What are the treatments? How could it have been prevented? The Diabetes Problem Solver is the first reference guide that helps you identify and prevent the most common diabetes-related problems you encounter from day to day. From hypoglycemia, nerve pain, and foot ulcers to eye disease, depression, and eating disorders, virtually every possible problem is covered. And the solutions are at your fingertips. The Diabetes Problem Solver addresses each problem by answering five crucial questions:

1. What are the symptoms?
2. What are the risks?

3. What do I do now?

4. What's the best treatment?

5. How can I prevent this problem?

You'll find extensive, easy-to-read coverage of just about every diabetes problem you can imagine, and comprehensive flowcharts at the front of the book lead you from symptoms to possible solutions quickly.

One Low Price: $19.95
Order #4825-01

New!

Diabetes Burnout: What to Do When You Can't Take It Anymore

William H. Polonsky, PhD, CDE

Living with diabetes is hard work. It's easy to get discouraged, frustrated and depressed—just plain old burned out. Finally there's a book that understands the roller-coaster of emotions you go through and gives you the tools you need to keep the "downers" from overwhelming you—all in a compassionate and even humorous way. It can help you pinpoint whether you've hit diabetes burnout (if so, you're not alone!).

One Low Price: $18.95
Order #4822-01

New!

16 Myths of a Diabetic Diet

Karen Hanson Chalmers, MS, RD, CDE
Amy E. Peterson, MS, RD, CDE

Now there's an easier way to debunk the myths you often hear such as "you need to eat foods sweetened with sugar substitutes instead of sugar,""don't eat too many starchy foods," and "no snacking or giving in to food cravings,"even that you have to eat different food from everyone else. This exciting book sets the record straight on the 16 most common myths about food and diet.

One Low Price: $14.95
Order #4829-01

New!

101 Foot Care Tips for People with Diabetes

Jessie H. Ahroni, PhD, ARNP, CDE

"Diabetic foot problems cause more hospital stays than any other complication of diabetes. This book tells you what to do for good foot care. It can help you stand on your own two feet for a lifetime!"
—Neil M. Schaffler, DPM, FACFAS
President, Baltimore Podiatry Group

- What should I do if I nick myself while trimming my toenails?
- How can I tell whether my shoes fit?
- What should I do if I have bunions?

These are just a few of the 101 questions answered in this indispensable new book for people with diabetes.

One Low Price: $14.95
Order #4834-01

101 Medication Tips for People with Diabetes

Betsy A. Carlisle, PharmD
Mary Anne Koda-Kimble, PharmD, CDE
Lisa Kroon, PharmD

1. What is the difference between regular and lispro insulin?
2. What are the main side effects of the drugs used to treat type 2 diabetes?
3. Will my diabetes medications interact with other drugs I'm taking?
4. My doctor prescribed an "ACE inhibitor." What is this drug? What will it do?

Treating diabetes can get complicated, especially when you consider the bewildering number of medications that must be carefully integrated with diet and exercise. Here you'll find answers to 101 of the most commonly asked questions about diabetes and medication. An indispensable reference for anyone with type 1, type 2, or gestational diabetes.

One Low Price: $14.95
Order #4833-01

101 Nutrition Tips for People with Diabetes

Patti B. Geil, MS, RD, FADA, CDE
Lea Ann Holzmeister, RD, CDE

1. Which type of fiber helps my blood sugar?

2. What do I do if my toddler refuses to eat her meal?

3. If a food is sugar-free, can I eat all I want?

In this latest addition to the best-selling 101 Tips series, co-authors Patti Geil and Lea Ann Holzmeister—experts on nutrition and diabetes—use their professional experience with hundreds of patients over the years to answer the most commonly asked questions about diabetes and nutrition. You'll discover handy tips on meal planning, general nutrition, managing medication and meals, shopping and cooking, weight loss, and more.

One Low Price: $14.95
Order #4828-01

Newly Revised!

101 Tips for Improving Your Blood Sugar, 2nd Edition

David S. Schade, MD, and The University of New Mexico Diabetes Care Team

Last night you ate a normal meal and took your usual insulin dose. When you woke up this morning you had low blood sugar. Why?

You work hard all week and you like to reward yourself by sleeping in on weekends. How can you avoid waking up with high blood sugar?

These are just a couple of the more than 100 tips you'll discover in this newly revised second edition of an ADA bestseller. Dozens of other tips—many of them just added—will help you reduce the risk of complications from extremes in blood sugar levels.

One Low Price: $14.95
Order #4805-01

Newly Revised!

101 Tips for Staying Healthy with Diabetes (& Avoiding Complications), 2nd Edition

David S. Schade, MD, and The University of New Mexico Diabetes Care Team

1. Is testing your urine for glucose and ketones an accurate way to measure blood sugar?

2. What's the best way to reduce the pain of frequent finger sticks?

3. Will an insulin pump help you prevent complications?

These are just a few of the more than 110 tips you'll discover in this newly revised second edition of an ADA bestseller. Dozens of other tips—many of them just added—will help you reduce the risk of complications and help you lead a healthy life.

One Low Price: $14.95
Order #4810-01

Diabetes Meal Planning on $7 a Day—or Less

Patti B. Geil, MS, RD, FADA, CDE
Tami A. Ross, RD, CDE

You can save money—lots of it—without sacrificing what's most important to you: a healthy variety of great-tasting meals. Learn how to save money by planning meals more carefully, use shopping tips to save money at the grocery store, eat at your favorite restaurants economically, and much more. Each of the 100 quick and easy recipes includes cost per serving and complete nutrition information to help you create a more cost-conscious, healthy meal plan.

One Low Price: $12.95
Order #4711-01

Meditations on Diabetes

Catherine Feste

Modern medicine has come full circle to realize again what ancient healers knew: that illness affects both the body and the soul. Cathy Feste has lived with diabetes for 40 years, so she knows the physical, emotional, and spiritual challenges that come with diabetes. With every turn of the page you'll discover reassuring advice and insight in daily meditations from the author's journals with a little help from her friends, such as Ralph Waldo Emerson, Eleanor Roosevelt, Helen Keller, and many others.

One Low Price: $13.95
Order #4820-01

When Diabetes Hits Home

Wendy Satin Rapaport, LCSW, PsyD

A reassuring exploration of the full spectrum of emotional issues you and your family may struggle with throughout your lives. You'll learn how to cope with the initial period of anger and anxiety at diagnosis, develop your spiritual self and discover the meaning of living with a chronic disease, address the changes all families go through and learn how to cope with them emotionally, and much more.

One Low Price: $19.95
Order #4818-01

The Uncomplicated Guide to Diabetes Complications

Edited by Marvin E. Levin, MD
and Michael A. Pfeifer, MD

Thorough, comprehensive chapters cover everything you need to know about preventing and treating diabetes complications—in simple language that anyone can understand. All major complications and special concerns are covered, including kidney disease, heart disease, obesity, eye disease and blindness, impotence and sexual disorders, hypertension and stroke, neuropathy and vascular disease, and more.

One Low Price: $18.95
Order #4814-01

The Dinosaur Tamer

Marcia Mazur and others

Enjoy 25 fictional stories that will entertain, enlighten, and ease your child's frustrations about having diabetes. Each tale warmly evaporates the fear of insulin shots, blood tests, and more. Ages 8–12.

Nonmember: $9.95
Member: $8.95
Order #4906-01

The Take-Charge Guide to Type I Diabetes

A guide written exclusively for people with Type 1 diabetes. Discover how to prevent or slow down complications, increase your chances of having a healthy baby, learn from testing your blood sugar, and much more.

Nonmember: $16.95
Member: $14.95
Order 4806-01

Winning with Diabetes

Inspiring true stories of people who live life to the fullest, despite having diabetes.

One Low Price: $12.95
Order #4824-01

Dear Diabetes Advisor

Michael A. Pfeifer, MD, CDE

Solid, no-nonsense answers to commonsense questions about diabetes.

Nonmember: $9.95
Member: $8.95
Order #4813-01

The Ten Keys to Helping Your Child Grow Up with Diabetes

Tim Wysocki, PhD

Here's help for parents who face the bewildering problems, feelings, and situations that can accompany all involved with diabetes, and the unpredictable emotional forces: depression, anger, guilt, and more.

Nonmember: $14.95
Member: $13.95
Order #4908-01

Commonsense Guide to Weight Loss

Barbara Caleen Hansen, PhD
Shauna S. Roberts, PhD

Learn how to lose weight—and keep it off—using medically proven techniques from the weight-loss experts. You'll discover the seven crucial elements of weight loss for people with diabetes, including how to choose the right target weight; make permanent lifestyle changes; measure weight-loss progress by tracking health, not weight; develop a healthy meal plan; maintain an active lifestyle and more.

One Low Price: $19.95
Order #4816-01

Complete Weight Loss Workbook

Judith Wylie-Rosett, EdD, RD
Charles Swencionis, PhD
Arlene Caban, BS
Allison J. Friedler, BS
Nicole Schaffer, MA

Proven techniques for controlling weight-related health problems. The authors devised a unique workbook that offers a series of checklists, worksheets, mini-cases, calculation exercises, mental reminders, and other practical aids to knocking off those extra pounds and staying fit for good. Features real-life examples of people who illustrate and explain the patterns that lead to success or failure in watching your weight.

One Low Price: $17.95
Order #4812-01

Bestseller!

Diabetes & Pregnancy

Learn about an unborn baby's development, tests to expect, labor and delivery and more.

Nonmember: $9.95
Member: $8.95
Order #4903-01

Cooking and Nutrition

New!

More Diabetic Meals in 30 Minutes—or Less!

Robyn Webb

Robyn Webb is back weaving her magic in your kitchen! She's whipped up hundreds more simply sensational recipes from mouth watering appetizers and succulent seafood dishes to tantalizing desserts. Choose from any of 225 fabulous recipes that not only satisfy your appetite and your carvings and taste savory and delicious but also meet ADA nutritional guidelines.

Each recipe gives you nutritional content and exchanges as well as fat and calorie counts.

One Low Price: $16.95
Order #4629-01

The Great Chicken Cookbook for People with Diabetes

Beryl M. Marton

Now you can have chicken any way you want it—and healthy too! More than 150 great-tasting, low-fat chicken recipes in all, including baked chicken, braised chicken, chicken casseroles, grilled chicken, rolled and stuffed chicken, chicken soups, chicken stir-fry, chicken with pasta, and many more.

One Low Price: $16.95
Order #4627-01

The New Soul Food Cookbook for People with Diabetes

Fabiola Demps Gaines, RD, LD
Roniece Weaver, RD, LD

Dig into sensational low-fat recipes from the first African American cookbook for people with diabetes. More than 150 recipes in all, including Shrimp Jambalaya, Fried Okra, Orange Sweet Potatoes, Corn Muffins, Apple Crisp, and many more.

One Low Price: $14.95
Order #4623-01

The Diabetes Snack Munch Nibble Nosh Book

Ruth Glick

Choose from 150 low-sodium, low-fat snacks and mini-meals such as Pizza Puffs, Mustard Pretzels, Apple-Cranberry Turnovers, Bread Puzzle, Cinnamon Biscuits, Pecan Buns, Alphabet Letters, Banana

Pops, and many others. Special features include recipes for one or two and snack ideas for hard-to-please kids. Nutrient analyses, preparation times, and exchanges are included with every recipe.

One Low Price: $14.95
Order #4622-01

The ADA Guide to Healthy Restaurant Eating

Hope S. Warshaw, MMSc, RD, CDE

Finally! One book with all the facts you need to eat out intelligently— whether you're enjoying burgers, pizza, bagels, pasta, or burritos at your favorite restaurant. Special features include more than 2,500 menu items from more than 50 major restaurant chains, complete nutrition information for every menu item, restaurant pitfalls and strategies for defensive restaurant dining and much more.

One Low Price: $13.95
Order #4819-01

Quick & Easy Diabetic Recipes for One

Kathleen Stanley, CDE, RD, MSED
Connie C. Crawley, MS, RD, LD

More than 100 breakfast, lunch, dinner, and snack recipes cut down to single-serving size.

One Low Price: $12.95
Order #4621-01.

Month of Meals: Classic Cooking

Choose from the classic tastes of Chicken Cacciatore, Oven Fried Fish, Sloppy Joes, Shish Kabobs, Roast Leg of Lamb, Lasagna, Minestrone Soup, Grilled Cheese Sandwiches, amd many others. And just because it's Christmas doesn't mean you have to abandon your healthy meal plan. A Special Occasion section offers tips for brunches, holidays, parties, and restaurants to give you delicious dining options in any setting. 58 pages. Spiral-bound.

One Low Price: $14.95
Order #4701-01

Month of Meals: Ethnic Delights

A healthy diet doesn't have to keep you from enjoying your favorite restaurants: tips for Mexican, Italian, and Chinese restaurants are featured. Quick-to-fix and ethnic recipes are also included. Choose from Beef Burritos, Chop Suey, Veal Piccata, Stuffed Peppers, and many others. 63 pages. Spiral-bound.

One Low Price: $14.95
Order #4702-01

Month of Meals: Meals in Minutes

Eat at McDonald's, Wendy's, Taco Bell, and other fast food restaurants and still maintain a healthy diet. Special sections offer tips on planning meals when you're ill, reading ingredient labels, preparing for picnics and barbecues, more. Quick-to-fix menu choices include Seafood Stir Fry, Fajita in a Pita, Hurry-Up Beef Stew, Quick Homemade Raisin Bread, Macaroni and Cheese, many others. 80 pages. Spiral-bound.

One Low Price: $14.95
#4703-01

Month of Meals: Old-Time Favorites

Old-time family favorites like Meatloaf and Pot Roast will remind you of the irresistible meals grandma used to make. Hints for turning family-size meals into delicious "planned-overs" will keep leftovers from going to waste. Meal plans for one or two people are also featured. Choose from Oven Crispy Chicken, Beef Stroganoff, Kielbasa and Sauerkraut, Sausage and Cornbread Pie, and many others. 74 pages. Spiral-bound.

One Low Price: $14.95
Order #4704-01

Month of Meals: Vegetarian Pleasures

Choose from a garden of fresh selections like Eggplant Italian, Stuffed Zucchini, Cucumbers with Dill Dressing, Vegetable Lasagna, and many others. Craving a snack? Try Red Pepper Dip, Eggplant Caviar, or Beanito Spread. A special section shows you the most nutritious ways to cook with whole grains, and how to add flavor to your meals with peanuts, walnuts, pecans, pumpkin seeds, and more. 58 pages. Spiral-bound.

One Low Price: $14.95
Order #4705-01

Official Pocket Guide to Diabetic Exchanges

Finally! A pocket-sized version of ADA's most popular aid to balanced nutrition.

Nonmember: $5.95
Member: $4.95
Order #4709-01

The Diabetes Carbohydrate & Fat Gram Guide, 2nd Edition

Lea Ann Holzmeister, RD, CDE

Hundreds of charts list foods, serving sizes, and nutrient data for generic and packaged products.

One Low Price: $14.95
Order #4708-02

Brand-Name Diabetic Meals in Minutes

More than 200 kitchen-tested recipes from Swanson, Campbell Soup, Kraft Foods, and more.

Nonmember: $12.50
Member: $9.95
Order #4620-01

Complete Quick & Hearty Cookbook

Features dozens of simple yet delicious recipes from the best of the popular Healthy Selects cookbook series.

One Low Price: $12.95
Order #4624-01

Bestseller!

Diabetic Meals in 30 Minutes—or Less!

Robyn Webb

Choose from more than 140 delicious, quick-to-fix meals from best-selling author Robyn Webb.

Nonmember: $11.95
Member: $9.95
Order #4614-01

Bestseller!

Diabetes Meal Planning Made Easy, 2nd Edition

Hope S. Warshaw, MMSc, RD, CDE

Discover how to master the food pyramid, understand Nutrition Facts and food labels, more.

Member: $14.95
Nonmember: $11.95
Order #4706-02

Magic Menus

Spanish Omelets, Blueberry Muffins, Oven-Fried Chicken, Caesar Salad, more.

Nonmember: $14.95
Member: $12.95
Order #4707-01

Memorable Menus

Robyn Webb

Roast Turkey Tenderloins, Honey-Mustard Chicken, Southern Shrimp Gumbo, more.

Nonmember: $19.95
Member: $17.95
Order #4619-01

Sweet Kids

Betty Page Brackenridge, MS, RD, CDE
Richard R. Rubin, PhD, CDE

Practical meal planning and nutrition advice for parents of diabetic children.

Nonmember: $11.95
Member: $9.95
Order #4905-01

Order Toll-Free: 1-800-232-6733

About the Authors

The authors are both mothers, work together at Children's Hospital of Pittsburgh, and have been friends for many years. *Raising a Child with Diabetes* is their second book for the American Diabetes Association.

Linda M. Siminerio, RN, PhD, CDE, has worked with children with diabetes for more than 25 years as a diabetes educator. She received a bachelor's degree in nursing from Pennsylvania State University, a master's degree in child development and childcare from the University of Pittsburgh, and a doctoral degree in health education from Pennsylvania State University. Her doctoral research was in diabetes education in pediatric populations. Dr. Siminerio is an active volunteer, past officer, and editor for the American Diabetes Association. She represents diabetes education for the International Diabetes Federation. Dr. Siminerio is an assistant professor and the Director of the Diabetes Institute at the University of Pittsburgh.

Jean Betschart, MN, MSN, CPNP, CDE, is a pediatric nurse practitioner and has been a diabetes educator since 1980. She has a bachelor's degree in nursing from the University of Pittsburgh, a master's degree in the nursing care of children, and a master's degree from the Department of Health Promotion and Development as a pediatric nurse practitioner. She was named Outstanding Health Professional Educator in 1994 by the American Diabetes Association. She is a past president of the American Association of Diabetes Educators and has volunteered for the American Diabetes Association at local, state, and national levels. She has written many books and articles for children with diabetes and their parents. Ms. Betschart developed type 1 diabetes during late adolescence.

About the American Diabetes Association

The American Diabetes Association is the nation's leading voluntary health organization supporting diabetes research, information, and advocacy. Its mission is to prevent and cure diabetes and to improve the lives of all people affected by diabetes. The American Diabetes Association is the leading publisher of comprehensive diabetes information. Its huge library of practical and authoritative books for people with diabetes covers every aspect of self-care—cooking and nutrition, fitness, weight control, medications, complications, emotional issues, and general self-care.

To order American Diabetes Association books: Call 1-800-232-6733. http://store. diabetes.org [Note: there is no need to use **www** when typing this particular Web address]

To join the American Diabetes Association:
Call 1-800-806-7801. www.diabetes.org/membership

For more information about diabetes or ADA programs and services:
Call 1-800-342-2383. E-mail: Customerservice@diabetes.org www.diabetes.org

To locate an ADA/NCQA Recognized Provider of quality diabetes care in your area: Call 1-703-549-1500 ext. 2202.
www.diabetes.org/recognition/Physicians/ListAll.asp

To find an ADA Recognized Education Program in your area:
Call 1-888-232-0822. www.diabetes.org/recognition/education.asp

To join the fight to increase funding for diabetes research, end discrimination, and improve insurance coverage: Call 1-800-342-2383. www.diabetes.org/advocacy

To find out how you can get involved with the programs in your community: Call 1-800-342-2383. See below for program Web addresses.

- *American Diabetes Month:* Educational activities aimed at those diagnosed with diabetes—month of November. www.diabetes.org/ADM
- *American Diabetes Alert:* Annual public awareness campaign to find the undiagnosed—held the fourth Tuesday in March. www.diabetes.org/alert
- *The Diabetes Assistance & Resources Program (DAR):* diabetes awareness program targeted to the Latino community. www.diabetes.org/DAR
- *African American Program:* diabetes awareness program targeted to the African American community. www.diabetes.org/africanamerican
- *Awakening the Spirit: Pathways to Diabetes Prevention & Control:* diabetes awareness program targeted to the Native American community. www.diabetes.org/awakening

To find out about an important research project regarding type 2 diabetes:
www.diabetes.org/ada/research.asp

To obtain information on making a planned gift or charitable bequest:
Call 1-888-700-7029. www.diabetes.org/ada/plan.asp

To make a donation or memorial contribution:
Call 1-800-342-2383. www.diabetes.org/ada/cont.asp

WITHDRAWAL